BLOOD FILTRATION AND BLOOD CELL DEFORMABILITY

DEVELOPMENTS IN HEMATOLOGY AND IMMUNOLOGY

Lijnen, H.R., Collen, D. and Verstraete, M., eds: Synthetic Substrates in Clinical Blood Coagulation Assays. 1980. ISBN 90-247-2409-0

Smit Sibinga, C.Th., Das, P.C. and Forfar, J.O., eds: Paediatrics and Blood Transfusion. 1982. ISBN 90-247-2619-0

Fabris, N., ed: Immunology and Ageing. 1982. ISBN 90-247-2640-9

Hornstra, G.: Dietary Fats, Prostanoids and Arterial Thrombosis. 1982. ISBN 90-247-2667-0

Smit Sibinga, C.Th., Das, P.C. and Loghem, van J.J., eds: Blood Transfusion and Problems of Bleeding. 1982. ISBN 90-247-3058-9

Dormandy, J., ed: Red Cell Deformability and Filterability. 1983. ISBN 0-89838-578-4

Smit Sibinga, C.Th., Das, P.C. and Taswell, H.F., eds: Quality Assurance in Blood Banking and Its Clinical Impact. 1984. ISBN 0-89838-618-7

Besselaar, A.M.H.P. van den, Gralnick, H.R. and Lewis, S.M., eds: Thromboplastin Calibration and Oral Anticoagulant Control. 1984. ISBN 0-89838-637-3

Fondu, P. and Thijs, O., eds: Haemostatic Failure in Liver Disease. 1984. ISBN 0-89838-640-3

Smit Sibinga, C.Th., Das, P.C. and Opelz, G., eds: Transplantation and Blood Transfusion. 1984. ISBN 0-89838-686-1

Schmid-Schönbein, H., Wurzinger, L.J. and Zimmerman, R.E., eds: Enzyme Activation in Blood-Perfused Artificial Organs. 1985. ISBN 0-89838-704-3

Dormandy, J., ed: Blood Filtration and Blood Cell Deformability. 1985. ISBN 0-89838-714-0

Blood Filtration and Blood Cell Deformability

Summary of the proceedings of the third workshop held in London, 6 and 7 October 1983, under the auspices of the Royal Society of Medicine and the Groupe de Travail sur la Filtration Erythrocytaire

edited by

JOHN DORMANDY, M.D., F.R.C.S.

St. James' and St. George's Hospitals
London

1985 **MARTINUS NIJHOFF PUBLISHERS**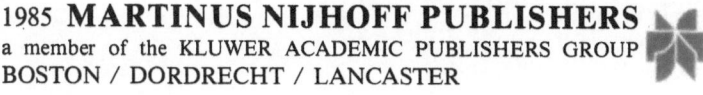
a member of the KLUWER ACADEMIC PUBLISHERS GROUP
BOSTON / DORDRECHT / LANCASTER

Distributors

for the United States and Canada: Kluwer Academic Publishers, 190 Old Derby Street, Hingham, MA 02043, USA
for the UK and Ireland: Kluwer Academic Publishers, MTP Press Limited, Falcon House, Queen Square, Lancaster LA1 1RN, UK
for all other countries: Kluwer Academic Publishers Group, Distribution Center, P.O. Box 322, 3300 AH Dordrecht, The Netherlands

Library of Congress Cataloging in Publication Data

Main entry under title:

Blood filtration and blood cell deformability.

  (Developments in hematology and immunology)
  Bibliography: p.
  1. Blood cells--Deformability--Congresses.
2. Erythrocytes--Deformability--Congresses. 3. Blood
cells--Congresses. 4. Blood--Filtration--Congresses.
4. Blood--Filtration--Congresses. I. Dormandy, J. A.
II. Royal Society of Medicine (Great Britain)
III. Groupe de travail sur la filtration erythrocytaire
(France) IV. Series. [DNLM: 1. Erythrocyte
Deformability--congresses. 2. Erythrocytes--physiology--
congresses. 3. Leukocytes--physiology--congresses.
4. Ultrafiltration--methods--congresses.
W1 DE997VZK / WH 150 B6548 1983]
QP96.B55 1985   612'.111   85-8941

ISBN-13: 978-0-89838-714-8   e-ISBN-13: 978-94-009-5008-5
DOI: 10.1007/978-94-009-5008-5

Copyright

Contents

List of participants   IX

Introduction and welcome by J.A. Dormandy   1

Welcome on behalf of the groupe de travail sur la filtration erythrocytaire by G.A. Marcel   3

The place of red cell filterability in the microcirculation by P. Gaehtgens   5

Effect of white blood cells on red cell filterability and the measurement of red cell deformability

Effect of white blood cells on red cell filterability by R. Skalak   13

Filterability of leucocyte suspensions by S. Chien   15

Effects of white blood cells in filtration measurements by M. Hanss   17

Qualitative and quantitative effects of white blood cells in a positive-pressure filtration system by G.D.O. Lowe   18

Effect of contaminating leucocytes on erythrocyte filterability by J. Stuart   20

Non-white cell clogging by J.A. Dormandy   23

Summary by H.J. Meiselman   25

Preparation of blood samples for filtration studies

Anticoagulant effects on the measurement of erythrocyte filterability by J. Stuart and I. Juhan-Vague   29

Effect of time delay from venepuncture on red cell rheology by A.J. Barnes   34

Red cell age distribution in blood centrifuged to remove leucocytes by M.Hanss   36

Erythrocyte volume stability in selected iso-osmotic buffers by H.J. Meiselman   37

Influence of the suspending medium on red blood cell filtration by S. Coccheri   41

Summary by J. Stuart   43

Comparison of different filtration techniques
Summary by G.A. Marcel   45

Comparison of blood filtration systems with other techniques for assessing red cell deformability

Comparison of red blood cell geometric and viscoelastic properties with various assays of red blood cell deformability: A preliminary analysis by H.J. Meiselman   55

Flow techniques and other devices for studying the distribution of the mechanical properties of red blood cells by J-C. Healy and P. Rusch   58

Comparison of filtration, micropipette aspiration and viscometry in osmotically swollen red blood cells by S. Chien   61

Comparison of whole blood filtration with three other methods of assessing red cell rheology in diabetics by A.J. Barnes   63

Preliminary report on the use of a new reusable metallic filter membrane by H. Schmid-Schönbein   65

Comparison of different types of filters with the use of erythrocytes with artificially bridged membranes by P. Teitel   66

New evidence on possible clinical relevance of blood filtration systems

Whole blood filtration in diabetes: What is its clinical meaning? by A.J. Barnes   71

Clinical relevance of the Siena technique by F. Laghi Pasini   73

Prognostic significance of whole blood filtration test in patients with cerebral infarction by M.R. Boisseau   75

Summary by J.A. Dormandy   76

The best feasible protocol for investigating the clinical effect of a haemorheological agent in leg ischaemia by S. Chien, J.A. Dormandy and R. Skalak   78

Classified biobliography prepared by G.D.O. Lowe   85

Commentary by M. Verstraete   99

Concluding remarks by P. Gaehtgens   101

List of participants

Dr Adrian Barnes
Barnet General Hospital, Wellhouse Lane, Barnet EN5 3DJ, UK

Professor Michel Boisseau
Hopital du Haut Leveque, Laboratoire d'Hematologie, Avenue de Magellan, 33600 Pessac, France

Professor Shu Chien
Physiology Department, Columbia University College of Physicians and Surgeons, 630 S. 168th Street, New York, USA

Professor Sergio Coccheri
Director, Department of Angiology & Blood Coagulation, University Hospital, Bologna, Italy

Mr John Dormandy
St James' Hospital, Sarsfeld Road, London SW12 8HW, UK

Professor Peter Gaehtgens
Freie Universität Berlin, Arminallee 22, D-1000 Berlin 33

Professor Maxime Hanss
Université Paris Nord, UER Experimentale, 74 Rue Marcel Cachin, 9300 Bobigny, France

Professor J-C. Healy
U.E.R. de Medicine, Laboratoire Biophysique et d'Informatique Medicale, 42023 Saint-Etienne, France

Dr Irène Juhan-Vague
Laboratoire Central d'Hématologie, Hôpital de la Timoni, 13385 Marseille, France

Dr Franco Laghi Pasini
Istituto di Patologia Speciale Medica, Universita di Siena, Istituti Clinici, Viale Bracci, 53100 Siena, Italy

X

Professor Pierre Leblond
Department of Medicine, Hospital du Saint-Sacrement, 1050 Chemin Ste-Foy, Quebec G1S 4L8, Canada

DrGordon Lowe
Department of Medicine, Glasgow Royal Infirmary, Glasgow G4 OSF, UK

Dr Georges Marcel
Laboratoires Hoechst, 3 Av. du General de Gaulle, 92800 Puteaux, France

Professor Herbert Meiselman
USC School of Medicine, 2025 Zonal Avenue (126 Mudd), Los Angeles, CA 90033, USA

Professor Holger Schmid-Schönbein
Abteilung Physiologie, Medizinische Fakultät, Rheinisch-Westfälische Technische Hochschule, Neuklinikum, Forckenbeckstrasse, Aachen, Federal Republic of Germany

Professor Richard Skalak
Bioengineering Institute, Columbia University, 610 Seeley W. Mudd Building, New York, NY 10027, USA

Professor John Stuart
Department of Haematology, The Medical School, Vincent Drive, Birmingham B15 2TJ, UK

Profesor Paul Teitel
Physiology Department, Rheinisch-Westfälische Technische Hochschule, Neuklinikum, Forckenbeckstrasse, Aachen, Federal Republic of Germany

Professor Marc Verstraete
Department of Medical Rearch, Campus Gasthuisberg, Herestraat 49, B-3000 Leuven, Belgium

Introduction and welcome

The proceedings of the Second Workshop on Red Cell Deformability and Filterability in 1982 were published almost verbatim and hopefully gave a vivid and complete picture of the state of the art at that time (Martinus Nijhoff, 1983). The orientation and membership of the Third Workshop in 1983 was slightly different, with increasing shift of emphasis from the red to the white cells. It was decided that on this occasion the published proceedings should take the form of a smaller update made up of a series of summaries by the participants. These have taken the form of surveys of whole areas of discussion, summaries of specific studies and two general commentaries by Professors Gaehtgens and Verstraete. Most references have been eliminated from these contributions and replaced by a general bibliography of the field of blood filtration prepared by Dr Lowe.

Hopefully researchers in this area will find this volume as useful and interesting as the previous published proceedings. The next meeting of the Workshop will probably take place in 1985 and will continue the changing interest towards white cell rheology. Again, I will be delighted to hear from any workers who have new data bearing on this topic.

J.A. Dormandy

Welcome on behalf of the Groupe de Travail sur la Filtration Erythrocytaire

G.A. Marcel

First of all, on behalf of the French Group, I would like to welcome all of our usual colleagues and also the newcomers. This is a slowly increasing ring. We have been in this room for quite a few years now. It is in this room that we started with John Dormandy preparing the London international conference, and there is already quite a lot of history here: we are already keeping to the same seats year after year! I very much enjoy these informal meetings. I think they are essential to the progress of our discipline and I sincerely hope that they will be able to go on for very many years. I think these informal scientific meetings, with no treasurer, vice-treasurer, sub-chairman and chairman are important because the only thing we are thinking about here is what these little cells are doing when they are going through filter pores and we do not have other problems obscuring our minds.

After these general philosophical words and these words of welcome, I would like to give special thanks to Professor Marc Verstraete for agreeing to come here. I have the luck to have known Professor Verstraete for a number of years and he has always been to me the symbol of both knowledge and the rigour in understanding. I think it is very important that we should have here an observer from what is practically a parallel field, although perhaps it encompasses it: the field of haemostasis and thrombosis. What we are working with certainly has a lot to do with haemostatis and thrombosis and also a lot to do with other fields, and I think it will be extremely interesting for us at the end of this meeting to have the unbiased view of such an observer on the discipline in which we are all working.

One last word of great thanks to the man who really organises all this, who does all the hard work – John Dormandy, thank you very much.

The place of red cell filterability in the microcirculation

P. Gaehtgens

This presentation is meant to provide a survey of the available data from which predictions of the relevance for the microcirculation of altered red cell properties detected by filterability measurements can be derived. It is obvious that the efforts undertaken to quantitatively determine this property of the erythrocytes have been considerable and not entirely unsuccessful. Yet, the concept which has prompted these efforts may from time to time require some re-evaluation.

It has long been well-known that red cells are indeed greatly deformed during passage through the microcirculation. This observation has more or less automatically led to the assumption that a loss of their ability to deform will result in a hemodynamic disturbance of the capillary circulation, an assumption which was supported by the fact that in many organs, notably skeletal or cardiac muscle and brain, capillary diameters tend to be smaller than the resting diameter of the circulating red cells, such that cell deformation is a prerequisite of capillary passage. Furthermore, studies of red cell 'deformability' by various in vitro methods have shown this property to be reduced in several diseases; such changes appeared to parallel an impairment of the microcirculation and were thus assumed to be a significant part of pathophysiology. However, the analysis of such correlations is complicated by the fact that in many diseases in which impaired red cell deformability has been found, other hemorheological changes (of red cell aggregation, plasma viscosity, leukocyte or platelet number or function) also occur: to my knowledge in none of these diseases has a loss of red cell deformability conclusively been shown to represent the only or even the most important *cause* of the disturbance. Mere observation of a microcirculatory disturbance does not suffice to identify the factors causing it. It is therefore very necessary to critically assess the evidence presented in favor of a concept which calls for a significant hemodynamic effect of altered red cell deformability in the living capillary circulation. In my view the problem here results from the fact that a simple mechanistic concept such as the effect of reduced deformability on capillary flow mechanics seems to be almost self-evident.

In actual fact, however, not much support can be drawn from the literature attempting to quantify in vivo the effect of alterations of red cell microrheology in general, and of alterations in deformability in particular. As examples I will only mention work done by LaCelle (1) or more recently by Driessen et al. (2), in which the attempt was made to measure flow velocities or resistance to flow in vessels of the microcirculation during perfusion with microrheologically altered red blood cells. These attempts have been rather unsuccessful in terms of the original concept: a demonstrable difference in flow velocity (and thus presumably flow resistance) could not be observed between normal red cells and sickle cells or spherocytes (1) or cells treated with diamide (2). It may be worth mentioning that according to Heast et al. (3) the survival rate even of glutaraldelyde fixed red cells in the circulation is not different from that of normal cells, at least within a time period of 4 hours. On the other hand, during perfusion of the capillary circulation with experimentally altered red cells, blockade of flow, particularly at capillary bifurcations was more often observed (1, 2, 4) than with normal red cells. However, no report seems to exist on the effect in vivo of the more subtle microrheological changes found in patients suffering from diseases other than sickle cell disease, or hereditary spherocytosis. The importance of deformability changes detectable in myocardial infarction, diabetes, or pheripheral vascular insufficiency has to my knowledge never been conclusively demonstrated in experiments in vivo, yet pathophysiological relevance is often attributed to such changes.

The situation being as it is, one could argue that changes of microrheology, be they as subtle as may be, are only *one* of many components of the pathophysiology of disease. Nevertheless, I tend to believe that we should urgently try to assess the importance of the phenomenon in vivo.

If at this stage in vivo evidence is missing, what is the *in vitro* evidence which might allow us to extrapolate to the living microcirculation?

In trying to assess the potential relevance, with respect to the living microcirculation, of changes in 'red cell filtrability' it may be useful to first define the microrheological events contributing to a filtration test. Previous discussion in this group has led to the conclusion that three phenomena must be expected to influence the result of a filtration measurement:

- the resistance incurring *during the passage* of single cells through a narrow pore,
- the effect of *cell entrance* into the narrow orifice of the pore, and
- the resistance changes resulting from *occlusion of pores* by cells unable to pass through.

We should try here to identify the correlates of these three phenomena in the living capillary circulation and in doing so also make use of data obtained in other in vitro systems.

The simplest case may be the complete *obstruction of pores*, either due to

WBC present (despite efforts to remove them) or to the presence of only a few rigid red cells. As mentioned above, in diseases leading to pronounced loss of 'deformability', occlusion of capillaries by red cells has been observed (sickle cells, hereditary spherocytes). Even the diamide-treated cells used by Driessen (2) seemed to occasionally block single capillaries, particularly at the site of bulging endothelial cells. Measurements of single pore passage time (6) seem also to show an increased rate of pore occlusion by diamide-treated or osmotically-treated cells. However, no evidence seems to have been reported that this phenomenon can be observed if the microrheology of the red cells is less artifically altered.

Increased resistance during cell passage through glass capillaries has been concluded from observations of prolonged transit times after isovolemic shape changes. Smooth spheres with presumably normal cell volume but reduced membrane surface areas as well as crenated spheres were shown to pass through 3–4 μm capillaries at significantly lower velocities than normal cells (5). Yet, on the other hand these observations are at odds with the findings in vivo reported above. It is amazing to see that the body of hard evidence even for an increased hydrodynamic resistance in straight tubes of capillary dimensions upon modification of 'cell deformability' is very scanty. Nevertheless, the possibility cannot be excluded that capillary resistance to cell passage may indeed be elevated if the ability of the red cells to deform is only moderately reduced (12). The discrepancy of data obtained by different methods (6) may also be a result of the different shearstress level employed in such studies. Incomplete recovery of capillary flow after a hypotensive period in vivo, but also the elevation of hydrodynamic resistance in vitro at very low pressure gradients observed by Driessen et al. (4) may indicate that no overt effect should be expected under 'normal' flow conditions, but may nevertheless occur under conditions of very low flow. This aspect, however, has not yet been systematically explored and extrapolations to the living microcirculation remain largely speculative.

Entrance effects have been studied in a variety of experimental models in vitro. Our own data (7) obtained by measuring the flux of red cells through narrow glass capillaries branching from a larger flow channel confirm earlier observations by Cokelet (8) by demonstrating a 'screening' effect: Even normal red cells tend to be partially excluded from the orifice of the capillary, if the forces diverting flow into the orifice are reduced (9). In very narrow capillaries (I.D. below 8 μm) this leads to significant cell exclusion. Hypertonic (600 mosm/l) shrinking of the cells with formation of echinocytes as well as (to a lesser degree) hypotonic (200 mosm/l) swelling resulted in intensified cell exclusion (7). In these studies an increase of flow resistance by approx. 10% associated with hypertonic shrinking was observed. From these observations, which have so far not been evaluated with patients' cells whose deformability is reduced, one might speculate that in vivo the heterogeneity of cell flux distribution and thus of the distribution of local oxygen delivery is increased. One could further speculate that this might lead to functional disturbances in the tissue affected, but more detailed studies must be carried out before this conclusion can be drawn.

Previous efforts of this group have led to an attempt to exclude cell–cell interaction from affecting a filtration measurement. Recent findings (10), however, suggest that this is only partially successful, and even aggregation effects cannot entirely be excluded if aggregation proteins are present in the suspending medium. Inasmuch as such phenomena must still be considered relevant, a change of cell–cell interactions following an alteration in single cell microrheology may also be considered to play a role in the microcirculation. Obviously, this will for dimensional reasons mainly be the case in the pre- or post-capillary vessels.

Application of data to the living microcirculation leads to the prediction of an increased loss of pressure energy in those vessels in which the shear stresses are the lowest: the venules. Increased venular resistance, in turn, must lead to elevated capillary pressures and/or reduction of total microvascular perfusion. While these changes may remain restricted both in quantitative terms and in their site of action under normal hemodynamic conditions, the entire range of microvessels, including arterioles, may be affected, if the arterio-venous driving pressures are lowered. The resulting elevation of viscous pressure dissipation in all microvessels must then inevitably result in significant flow reduction and thus impaired nutritive function of the microcirculation.

In summary then, I do not see sufficient evidence to predict whether and where the alteration of red cell microrheology detected by a filtration experiment will pose a significant threat to the living microcirculation. Aside from the absence of conclusive data demonstrating measurable effects directly in the capillaries, arterioles or venules, a thorough study not only of the correlation between red cell microrheology and the functional capacity of a potentially afflicted organ but also of the cause–effect relationship is badly needed. Extrapolation of hitherto available results suggests that it is not the capillary network alone which may be affected but also somewhat larger vessels, and this may be even more pronounced at low driving pressures. With the exception of but a few clinical diseases (possibly sickle cell disease, or certain hemolytic disorders) pathologically altered red cell rheology alone is unlikely to be operative in the manifestation of functional failure. The normal microcirculation may well be able to tolerate even significantly altered red cell mechanics, due to a variety of compensatory mechanisms such as vasodilator reserve, capillary recruitment, O_2-extraction reserve, etc. In all likelihood, it is only the microcirculation of the hemodynamically decompensated cardiovascular system which after exhaustion of these compensatory mechanisms may suffer additionally from flow-incompetent red blood cells. The conclusion, there-fore, must be that it is probably not even the poorly filterable red cell as such which is 'dangerous', but, at best, the combination of circumstances, hemo-dynamic, metabolic, and possibly rheological. In a setting of physiologic circumstances, even substantially rigidified erythrocytes might not by them-selves cause a threat to the microcirculation, yet in a setting of pathologic conditions they might contribute to cause adverse effects. We are, in my mind and at this time, far from being able to predict, in quantitative terms, the relative importance of red cell rheology in pathology.

References

1. La Celle, P.L. (1975). Blood *1*, 269–284.
2. Driessen, G.K. (1981). Habilitationsschrift, Rhein.-Westf. Techn. Hochschule Aachen.
3. Haest, C.W.M., Driessen, G.K., Kamp, D., Heidtmann, H., Fischer, T.M. and Stöhr-Liesen, M. (1980). Pflügers Arch., *388*, 69–73.
4. Driessen, G.K., Haest, C.W.M., Heidtmann, H., Kamp, D. and Schmid-Schönbein, H. (1980). Pflügers Arch., *388*, 75–78.
5. Braasch, D. (1971). Physiol. Rev., *51*, 679–701.
6. Kiesewetter, H., Dauer, U., Teitel, P., Schmid-Schönbein, H. and Trapp, R. (1982). Bio-rheology, *19*, 737–753.
7. Gaehtgens, P. (1981). Scand. J. clin. Lab. Invest., *41*, Suppl. 156, 83–87.
8. Cokelet, G.R. (1976). In: Microcirculation (Eds. J. Grayson, W. Zingg). New York, Plenum, Vol. 1, pp. 9–31.
9. Pries, A.R., Albrecht, K.H. and Gaehtgens, P. (1981). Biorheology, *18*, 355–367.
10. Schmid-Schönbein, H. (1983). In: Red Cell Deformability and Filterability (Ed. J. Dormandy. Boston, M. Nijhoff Publ., pp. 109–114.

Effect of white blood cells on red cell filterability and the measurement of red cell deformability

Introduction

At the 1982 Workshop on Red Cell Deformability and Filterability, several investigators presented data showing that white cells can have significant effects on the passage of either red cell–white cell suspensions or whole blood suspensions through filters and thus on the estimation of red cell deformability via filtration. The following short papers summarize the progress subsequently made by members of the Workshop in evaluating the specific effects of white cells on the red cell filtration process.

Effect of white blood cells on red cell filterability

R. Skalak

A macroscopic theory of the flow of a suspension of red and white blood cells through a nuclepore filter is given on the basis of the relative resistance β, which is the ratio of the resistance offered by a cell in flowing through a pore to the resistance of flow of the suspending fluid only. In previous theories, the resistance β of each cellular species was considered to be a constant. The theory has been expanded to include the possibility of a distribution of the β values for each cellular species. Normal distributions are used with a mean several times its standard deviation. Cells which plug pores are represented in this theory by high values of β. If a typical red blood cell has a β value of 5 and takes of the order of 10 milliseconds to traverse a pore, then a white blood cell with a resistance factor β of 1,000 will take approximately 2 seconds to traverse the filter.

The theory is based on equations of flow through each pore of the filter and the conservation of mass which leads to an accumulation of cells of high resistance in the filter. The present theory computes distributions of each species of cell in the filter at each time. It is shown that a transient curve of increasing pressure is produced by each species of cells present. The typical rise time of the pressure is several times the transit time of the cells through the filter. Thus, red blood cells reach an equilibrium distribution in the filter in a fraction of a second. White blood cells, which have a longer transit time, may take several seconds or minutes to reach an equilibrium. Generally, a small percentage of stiff white blood cells will gradually displace red blood cells in the filter and by their slow passage cause an increasing pressure with time.

Computations have also been carried out representing several species of white blood cells, paralleling experiments in which different white blood cells have been separated. As in the case of mixtures of red blood cells and white blood cells, when several species of white blood cells are present, the stiffest cells with high values of β may cause a gradual rise in pressure even if they are present in very small concentrations. Figure 1 shows the results of a computation assuming three species of cells are present with mean values of β of 100, 500, and 25,000 in concentrations of 0.1%, 0.1%, and 0.025. The uppermost

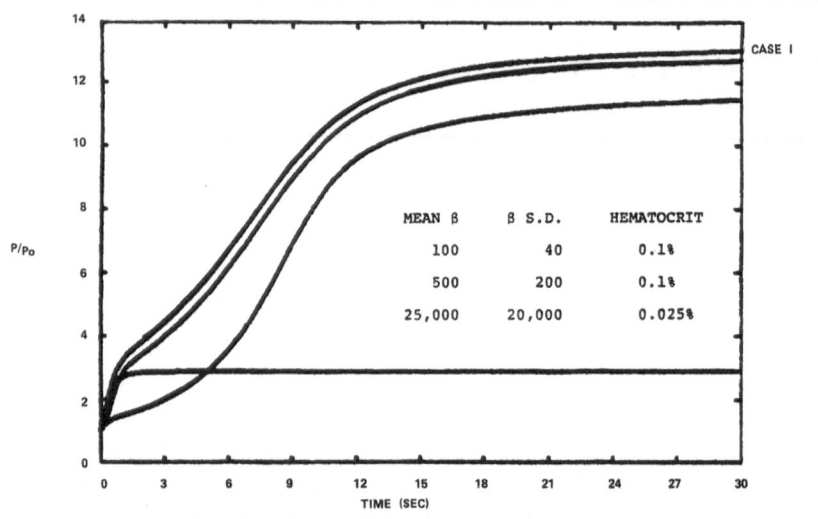

MEAN β	β S.D.	HEMATOCRIT
100	40	0.1%
500	200	0.1%
25,000	20,000	0.025%

CASE I

P/P₀

TIME (SEC)

Fig. 1. Case I.

curve shows the computed results with all three species present. The remaining curves show the results of removing the first, second, or third species. From these curves it is clear that the lower values of β cause a minor part of the long-term pressure rise observed; they contribute a relatively rapid transient which lasts about 2 or 3 seconds. The long-term (30 seconds) rise is only present when the stiffest cells are present, even though their concentration is only 0.025%. These computations indicate the main effect of white cells present in red blood cell suspensions in filterability testing. It is seen that even a small percentage of white blood cells present will determine the later time history of the pressure observed. The initial rapid transient rise of the pressure can be attributed to the most flexible components present; usually this will be the red cell fraction. The above discussion and accompanying curve apply to a case of constant discharge with a measurement of the pressure p as a function of time. The same theory can be used for pressure held constant so that flow will decrease with time, or a variable pressure or flow being specified.

Filterability of leucocyte suspensions

S. Chien

An application of the theory presented by Dr. Skalak on the filtration of a mixture of cells with different deformability is exemplified by some recent experiments performed by Dr. Emily Schmalzer and myself on the filterability of suspensions of leucocytes. Human leucocytes were separated by density into two fractions, one containing predominantly granulocytes (fraction I) and the other, lymphocytes and monocytes (fraction II). The filterability of these fractions and their mixture was determined by a constant-flow method through 5 μm Nuclepore filters, and the results are shown in Fig. 1. The pressure–time curve of fraction I indicates the behavior of a relatively homogeneous cell population. The pressure–time curve of fraction II can be analyzed to distinguish the effect of the more numerous and more deformable lymphocytes (early part) from the sparser but less deformable monocytes (later part). The pressure–time curve generated by the mixed leucocytes comprising both fractions exhibits the shape to be expected from such mix-

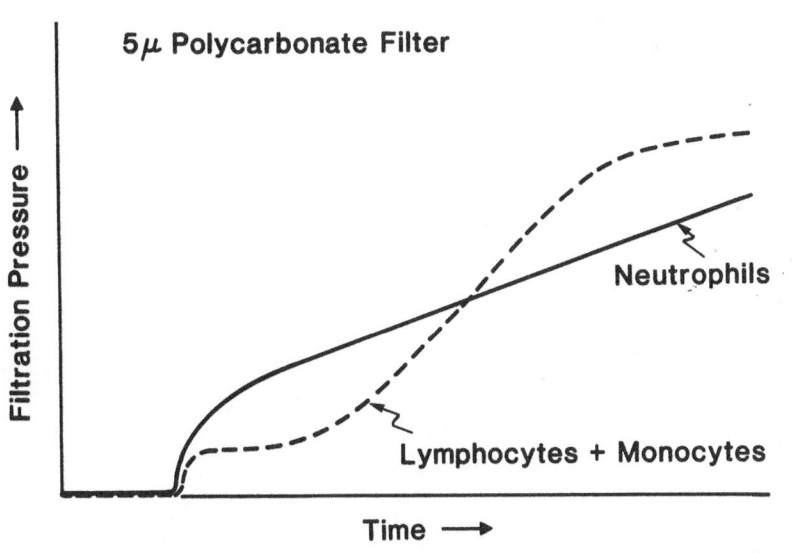

Fig. 1

tures. The pressure–time curves of the mixed leucocytes and fraction I were lowered by treating the cells with 1 and 10 mM of pentoxifylline (PTX). PTX did not affect the early part of the pressure–time curve for fraction II, but lowered the later part. These results suggest that PTX affects the deformability of the polymorphonuclear leucocytes and monocytes, but not the lymphocytes.

Effects of white blood cells in filtration measurements

M. Hanss

Recent reports have demonstrated that increasing the residual WBC count increased the filtration time of RBC suspensions. The clogging of the filter by the WBCs is the generally accepted explanation for this effect.

Let us consider a filtration experiment with the Hemorheometre technique. Typically, 50 to $100\,\mu l$ of a 8% (V/V) RBC suspension filters through the Nuclepore membrane in order to have a measurement. The number of available pores for the usual $5\,\mu m$ Nuclepore membranes is 10^5 ($4.10^5/cm^2$ pore density; about $0.4\,cm^2$ useful membrane area with the Hemorheometre). Therefore, about 100 RBCs filter through one average pore. With a normal WBC count (about 800 RBC for 1 WBC), only 1 pore out of 8 to 10 should then have the opportunity of being blocked or traversed by a WBC.

In filtration experiments, the WBC count is usually highly reduced (10 to 20 fold) so that usually less than 1 pore out of 100 is liable to blockage.

In conclusion, at a 1% accuracy level, the filtration time should not be affected by the mechanical pore blockage by WBCs. One way of reconciliating this conclusion and the reported results, is to propose indirect effects such as WBC–RBCs aggregate formation, or RBC stiffening through biochemical means due to the WBCs. In either case, the filtration time increase should positively correlate with the WBC count.

Qualitative and quantitative effects of white blood cells in a positive-pressure filtration system

G.D.O. Lowe

The presence of residual white cells in red cell suspensions complicates the interpretation of filtration tests for red cell deformability. One approach to this problem is to examine the *initial* pressure–flow relationship rather than the later part of the curve, since white cells progressively block the filter. Schmalzer and colleagues (Biorheology, 1983, *20*, 29–40) found no effect of suspension white cell concentration on the *initial* pressure of cell suspension relative to buffer, up to concentration $12 \times 10^9/l$. In a similar washed–cell positive pressure system (Nuclepore $5\,\mu$m filters, haematocrit 0.05, flow rate 1.5 ml/min) we have related suspension white cell count to both the initial pressure ratio (pi/Pb) as well as to the final pressure ratio after 6 minutes' filtration (Pf/Pb). Our standard washing procedure removes 90% of white

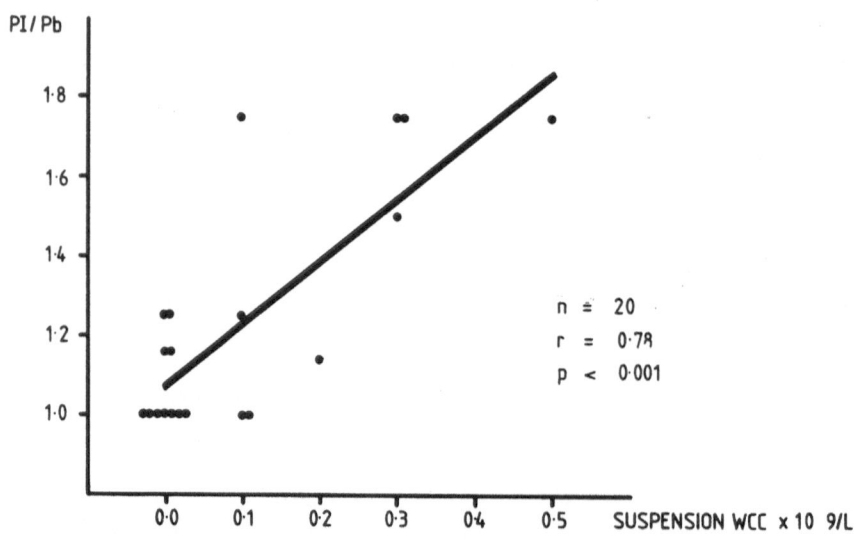

Fig. 1. Relationship of initial pressure ratio of cell suspension to buffer (Pi/Pb) to concentration of residual white cells in red cell suspensions (haematocrit 0.05).

cells on average, so at the time of the initial pressure reading we have on average only 1 white cell per 6000 red cells. However, unlike Schmalzer et al., we have found a significant relationship of the white cell concentration (range $0–0.5 \times 10^9/l$), not only to Pf/Pb, but also to Pi/Pb (Fig. 1). Thus, even at the start of filtration small numbers of residual white cells appear to influence the reading. Similar effects of white cells have also been reported using the Hémorhéomètre, which measures initial flow rate in a negative pressure system (G.S. Lucas et al., Clinical Hemorheology, in press). We conclude that in either type of Nuclepore filtration system, complete removal of white cells is necessary since even early readings are affected by small numbers of residual white cells.

We have also filtered pure red-cell-free suspensions of (a) polymorphs and (b) mononuclear cells (lymphocytes and monocytes), separated on a Ficoll-Hypaque density gradient. As expected, Pf/Pb increases strongly with increasing concentrations of both types of white cell. Within the range of residual white cells in our red cell suspensions, the influence of white cells alone on Pi/Pb appears insufficient to explain their effects in red cell suspensions simply in terms of white cell–pore interactions (Fig. 2) and this accords with Professor Hanss's calculations. Hence, one may postulate an effect of residual white cells on red cell passage: either mechanical 'crowding', or possibly a chemical effect as suggested by Professor Laghi Pasini and colleagues at this meeting.

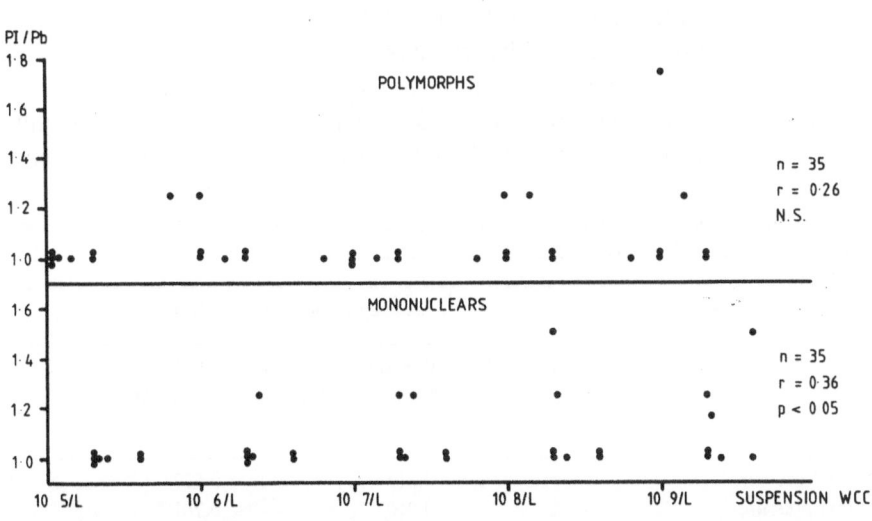

Fig. 2. Relationship of Pi/Pb to cell concentration in pure suspensions of polymorphs or mononuclear cells (haematocrit 0.00).

Effect of contaminating leucocytes on erythrocyte filterability

J. Stuart

Clinical studies from this department have convinced us of the effect of even small changes in blood leucocyte count on erythrocyte filterability. In diabetes mellitus (1), in normal pregnancy (2), and in clinical trials of drugs that alter the leucocyte count (3), we have found the results for positive-pressure erythrocyte filtration through the 5 μm diameter pores of polycarbonate membranes (Nuclepore) to be leucocyte dependent. Confirmation of this came from in vitro manipulation of the number of contaminating leucocytes in the test erythrocyte suspension to give residual leucocyte counts ranging from 0.08 to $1.6 \times 10^9/l$ and from 1.9 to $16.1 \times 10^9/l$ (4). Over both ranges a significant correlation (P<0.001) was found (Table 1) between the leucocyte count and all three methods of interpreting the positive-pressure time curves (initial pressure, final pressure, and the red cell filtration ratio). Thus, it was not possible to avoid leucocyte effects by removing some, but not all, leucocytes or by interpreting the pressure–time curves in a different way (4).

We had hoped that the initial-flow-rate (Hémorhéomètre) method (5) for measuring erythrocyte filterability would be leucocyte independent. Study of 36 erythrocyte test suspensions with the number of contaminating leucocytes adjusted to give a range from 0 to $1.0 \times 10^9/l$ showed, however, a highly significant correlation (r = 0.903; P<0.001) between residual leucocytes and

Table 1. Correlation (r) between three methods of interpreting positive-pressure time curves and the logarithm of the leucocyte count in the test cell suspension.

	Leucocyte count ($\times 10^9/l$) range	
	0.08–1.6 (25 specimens) r	1.9–16.1 (70 specimens) r
Initial pressure	0.812	0.577
Final pressure	0.910	0.701
Red cell filtration ratio	0.867	0.653

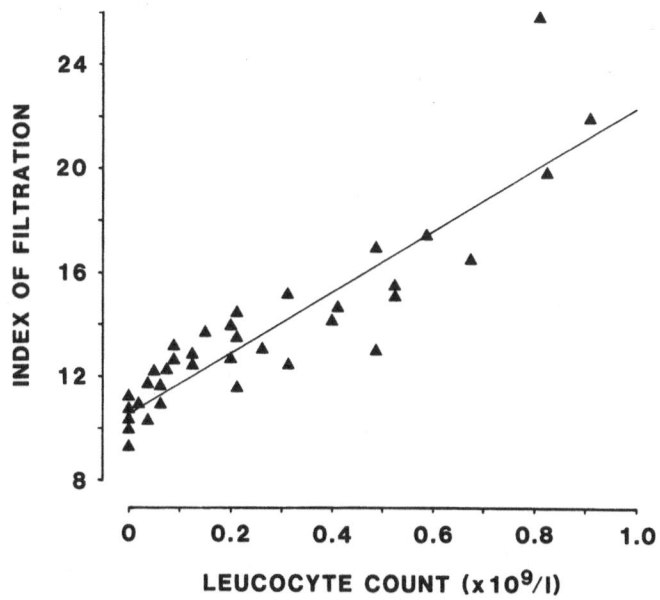

Fig. 1. Correlation between Hémorhéomètre index of filtration and the number of contaminating leucocytes in the test erythrocyte suspension. Calculated regression line shown for 36 test suspensions.

the index of filtration (6) using 5 μm pore diameter polycarbonate membranes (Fig. 1). Thus, since the initial-flow-rate gravity filtration method is also leucocyte dependent, there would seem to be no alternative to removing all contaminating leucocytes in order to obtain a true measurement of erythrocyte filterability.

References

1. Stuart, J., Kenny, M.W., Aukland, A., George, A.J., Neumann, V., Shapiro, L.M. and Cove, D.H. (1983). Filtration of washed erythrocytes in athero-sclerosis and diabetes mellitus. Clinical Hemorheology *3*, 23–30.
2. Stuart, J., Kenny, M.W. and Inglis, T.C.M. (1983). Erythrocyte filterability in normal pregnancy and pre-eclampsia. British Journal of Haematology, *53*, 353–355.
3. Neumann, V., Cove, D.H., Shapiro, L.M., George, A.J., Kenny, M.W., Meakin, M. and Stuart, J. (1983). Effect of Ticlopidine on platelet function and blood rheology in diabetes mellitus. Clinical Hemorheology, *3*, 13–21.
4. Kenny, M.W., Meakin, M. and Stuart, J. (1983). Methods for removal of leucocytes and platelets prior to study of erythrocyte deformability. Clinical Hemorheology, *3*, 191–200.
5. Hanss, M. (1983) Erythrocyte filtrability by the initial flow rate method. Biorheology, *20*, 199–211.

6. Lucas, G.S., Caldwell, N.M., Kenny, M.W., Meakin, M., Aillaud, M.F., Billerey, M., Juhan-Vague, I. and Stuart, J. (1983). Effect of calcium-chelating and non-chelating anticoagulants on erythrocyte and leucocyte filterability. Clinical Hemorheology, in press.

Non-white cell clogging

J. Dormandy

It has been found that even filtration techniques using buffy coat depleted cell resuspensions (e.g. Dodds-Dormandy technique) are affected by residual white cells. To study the clogging we used our new constant pressure filtration technique:

– *New constant pressure technique* (Matrai) detects changing flow rate so that the clogging rate and initial filtration rate can be determined independently. Fourty photoresistors are aligned at 4 mm intervals along a horizontal glass tube (I.D. 2 mm). A light beam is projected into the tube, and it is reflected by the retreating meniscus on to the photoresistors. The peak of the signal from each sensor is detected and the time interval between the peaks is measured electronically. The sample volume is 2.5 ml for each test. The progressive filter clogging results in a decrease of filter conductance. The initial filtration rate and the clogging rate can be determined from this plot. The method in its present state is too complex for routine use and we are now simplifying it to develop a cheap and reliable method to detect flow rate at constant pressure head. From the slope of the filter conductance versus volume filtered one can define the filter clogging as the relative decrease of the conductance per volume filtered, and the concentration of the plugging particles can be calculated.

Evidence for non-white cell clogging

Figure 1 shows the filter clogging determined by this method in reconstituted samples of five healthy subjects. Each group of symbols represents reconstituted samples of the same blood with different white cell counts. The straight line shows the ideal case when each white cell blocks one pore. The filter clogging correlates well with the white cell count; however there is a significant clogging for which the white cells cannot be responsible, even if all the white cells plugged a pore. This non-white cell clogging represents about 10^4–10^5 clogging particles per ml suspension in control samples of 0.05 haematocrit (red cell count = 5×10^8/ml).

Although it is generally accepted that whole blood filtration depends mainly

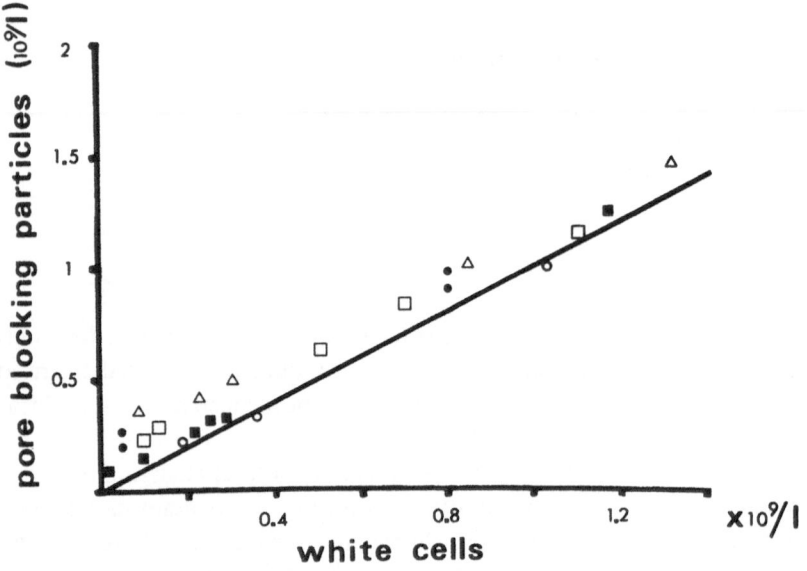

Fig. 1.

on white cell count, we believe that the total number of white cells does not account for all the observed differences. Presumably this non-white cell clogging, which may be due to very rigid red cells or aggregates, will become increasingly important as techniques are developed for removing the white cells completely.

Summary

H.J. Meiselman

From the theoretical studies of Dr. Skalak, it is clear that white cells can significantly influence the pressure–time profile of a red cell/white cell suspension, and that the presence of even a small amount of relatively rigid white cells can have a profound effect on the filtration pressure during the latter portion of a filtration experiment. Conversely, white cell effects, regardless of their relative rigidity, are shown to have only minimal effects during the very early (i.e., 0–2 seconds) phases of the filtration process. Dr. Chien's experimental data support these theoretical studies, in that white cells of different mechanical properties exhibit different pressure–time curves; pressure–time data for mixtures of leucocytes show shapes which can be predicted from the behavior of relatively homogeneous cell populations.

The insensitivity of the very early portions of the filtration process to white cells is again reflected in the calculations made by Dr. Hanss. Using the nominal dilutions, white cell concentrations and the total volume of filtered cell suspension, he indicates that usually less than 1 pore out of 100 is liable to blockage by white cells. He thus concludes that, at the 1% accuracy level, initial filtration data should not be affected by mechanical pore blockage by white cells.

Experimental studies by Dr. Lowe and Dr. Stuart question the WBC-insensitivity of the early portion of the filtration process. Using a constant flow system, Dr. Lowe demonstrates a significant correlation between the *initial* filtration pressure (reported as the ratio of initial pressure to cell-free buffer pressure) and white cell concentration over a white cell concentration range of 0 to 5×10^8 per liter. In addition, using red-cell-*free* white cell suspensions, there were only relatively minor effects on this initial pressure ratio for either polymorphs or mononuclear white cells; these effects in a red-cell-free suspension were not sufficient to explain the initial pressure which was observed when red cells were present. It is thus suggested by Dr. Lowe (and by Dr. Hanss) that the initial pressure effects of white cells may be due to a mechanical 'crowding' interaction between red and white cells or to more specific chemical effects in which the white cells induce either white cell–red cell aggregates or increased red cell rigidity.

The experimental results presented by Dr. Stuart involved studies using both positive pressure and initial flow rate filtration methods. In the former, significant white cell effects were observed for *all* three methods of interpreting the pressure–time curves; initial pressure as well as final pressure and red cell filtration ratio were effected for white cell concentrations of from 8×10^7 to 1.6×10^{10} per liter. The latter studies, using the Hanss Hemorheometre to obtain the initial flow rate of suspension, were *also* strongly influenced by white cells; the initial pressure increased in a linear fashion over a white cell concentration from 0 to 1.6×10^9 per liter. Thus, both Dr. Lowe and Dr. Stuart indicate that all filtration tests, even those measuring the initial flow rate, are leucocyte dependent and that there seems to be no alternative to removing all contaminating leucocytes in order to obtain a true measurement of erythrocyte filterability.

Non-white cell clogging of filter pores also appears to be an important aspect of the filtration process. Using his new constant-pressure filtration system, Mr. Dormandy indicates that even if one assumes that each white cell blocks one pore, there is a significant clogging for which white cells cannot be responsible. It is thus suggested that this non-white cell clogging phenomenon may be due to very rigid red cells or to aggregates, a view that is not in disagreement with the general suggestions of Drs. Hanss, Lowe and Stuart.

In overview, it is clear that white cells can influence all phases of the filtration process, even though theoretical considerations suggest significant effects only during the latter portions of filtration. Thus, there is a need to both extend the current analyses to account for these experimental observations and to continue the experimental work in order to define the possible mechanical and chemical interactions between red cells and white cells which give rise to these initial pressure or initial flow effects. In addition, the above material suggests at least two other areas in which work is needed: 1) examination of the filtration method as a possible tool for the measurement of white cell mechanical properties (deformability, filterability) in order to gain further insight into the rheologic behavior of these cells when flowing in small geometry pores; 2) a re-consideration of whole blood filtration studies as an index to the overall small-geometry flow behavior of the complete suspension, without trying to force a red cell mechanical property from the data obtained on a mixture of several cell types. Note that the following recent publications provide relevant information on white cell mechanical behavior and thus should be of value to those interested in white cell or white cell–red cell filtration: White Blood Cells, edited by U. Bagge, G.V.R. Born and P. Gaehtgens, M. Nijhoff Publishers, 1982; White Cell Mechanics, edited by H.J. Meiselman, M.A. Lichtman and P.L. La Celle, A.R. Liss, Inc., 1984.

Preparation of blood samples for filtration studies

Introduction

At the 1982 Workshop on Red Cell Deformability and Filterability, data were presented to show that the method used for storage and preparation of blood samples was an important variable in the subsequent measurement of erythrocyte deformability (filterability). The main factors were thought to be the anticoagulant used, time delay from venepuncture, storage temperature, and the buffer used to prepare the test erythrocyte suspension. The following short papers summarise the progress subsequently made by members of the Workshop in the development of improved methods for preparing blood samples for filtration studies.

Anticoagulant effects on the measurement of erythrocyte filterability

J. Stuart and I. Juhan-Vague

The data we presented at the 1982 Workshop indicated that erythrocyte deformability, as measured by positive-pressure filtration through 5 μm pore diameter polycarbonate (Nuclepore) membranes, was affected by the anticoagulant used during storage of the whole blood sample at room temperature (1). Subsequent analysis of the pressure–time curves of this system showed that the initial pressure (steady state slope of filtration curve extrapolated back to zero time; Pi) was the most sensitive of the curve parameters to these anticoagulant effects.

Twelve normal blood samples were therefore taken into K_2EDTA (1.5 mg/ml added blood; Seward Laboratory, UAC House, Blackfriars Road, London SE1 9UG) and stored for 6 hours at room temperature; there was no significant change in the mean Pi value with time (Fig. 1). When the same 12 bloods were taken into lithium heparin (15 IU/ml added blood; Sterilin Ltd., Teddington, Middlesex), there was a significantly lower (P<0.05) value for Pi (Fig. 1) at 1 h from venepuncture (heparin – mean 3.41, SEM 1.04; EDTA – mean 4.22, SEM 0.18). At 2 h and thereafter, the Pi values for heparinised blood had significantly increased so that there was no longer any significant difference from EDTA blood (Fig. 1). While this study (2, 3) showed an obvious difference between the two anticoagulants, it was not clear whether the difference reflected an anticoagulant effect on the filtered erythrocytes or on contaminating platelets or leucocytes.

We therefore studied the effect of storage of whole blood in EDTA and heparin on platelets and leucocytes. For EDTA samples, taken from 12 normal individuals, there was no significant change in mean platelet count over 6 h (Fig. 2) whereas 12 blood specimens taken into Vacutainer heparin (Becton Dickinson Vacutainer Systems, Rutherford, New Jersey, USA) showed thrombocytopenia (Fig. 2), which was a consequence of platelet microaggregate formation (2). It is known that heparin-induced platelet microaggregates can cause blockage of the 5 μm diameter pores of polycarbonate membranes (4).

Leucocytes were also found to be adversely affected by heparin in a time-

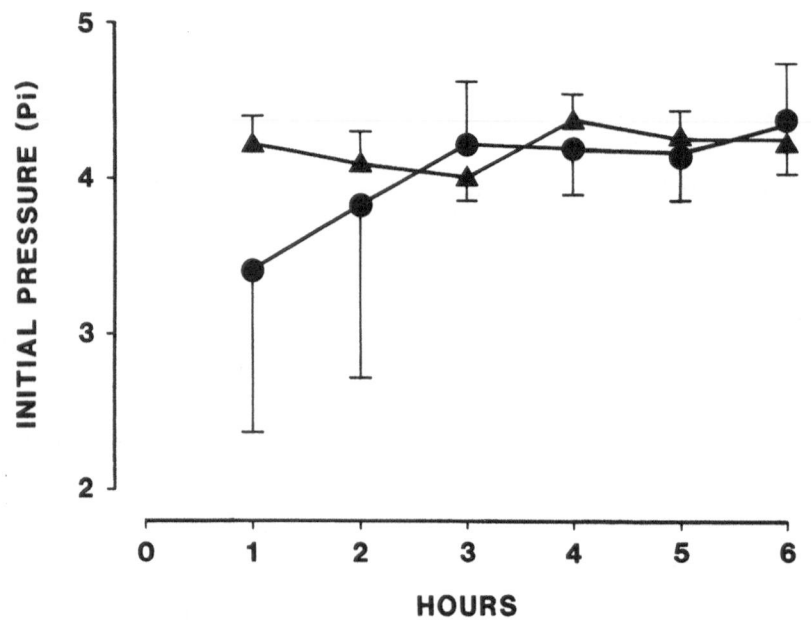

Fig. 1. Effect of storage of whole blood in EDTA (▲) and heparin (●) for up to 6 hours at room temperature on the initial pressure (Pi) of positive-pressure erythrocyte filtration.

dependent manner. Leucocytes stored in heparin at room temperature showed earlier morphological evidence of degeneration, such as cytoplasmic vacuolation, than did leucocytes taken into EDTA. Blood taken into Vacutainer heparin, but not EDTA, showed a progressive fall over 6 h in mean total leucocyte and absolute neutrophil counts, as determined by the Technicon Hemalog D system (Fig. 2). The neutrophil counting system of this instrument depends on myeloperoxidase cytochemical staining at 55° C and pH 3.2 which may have caused selective disruption of heparin-damaged neutrophils since visual leucocyte counts in a Neubauer chamber showed no significant leucopenia during 6 hours' storage in either EDTA or heparin.

Finally, we studied the positive-pressure filtration of washed erythrocyte suspensions enriched with leucocytes taken from autologous buffy coat preparations. At 3 h from venepuncture there was no change in filterability for blood originally taken into EDTA, whereas leucocyte-enriched erythrocyte suspensions prepared from heparinised blood showed 32–72% loss of filterability after 3 h (2). Heparin thus adversely affected leucocyte filterability in a time-dependent way.

For the above reasons, it is necessary to remove all contaminating platelets and leucocytes from erythrocyte test suspensions if the effects of anticoagu-

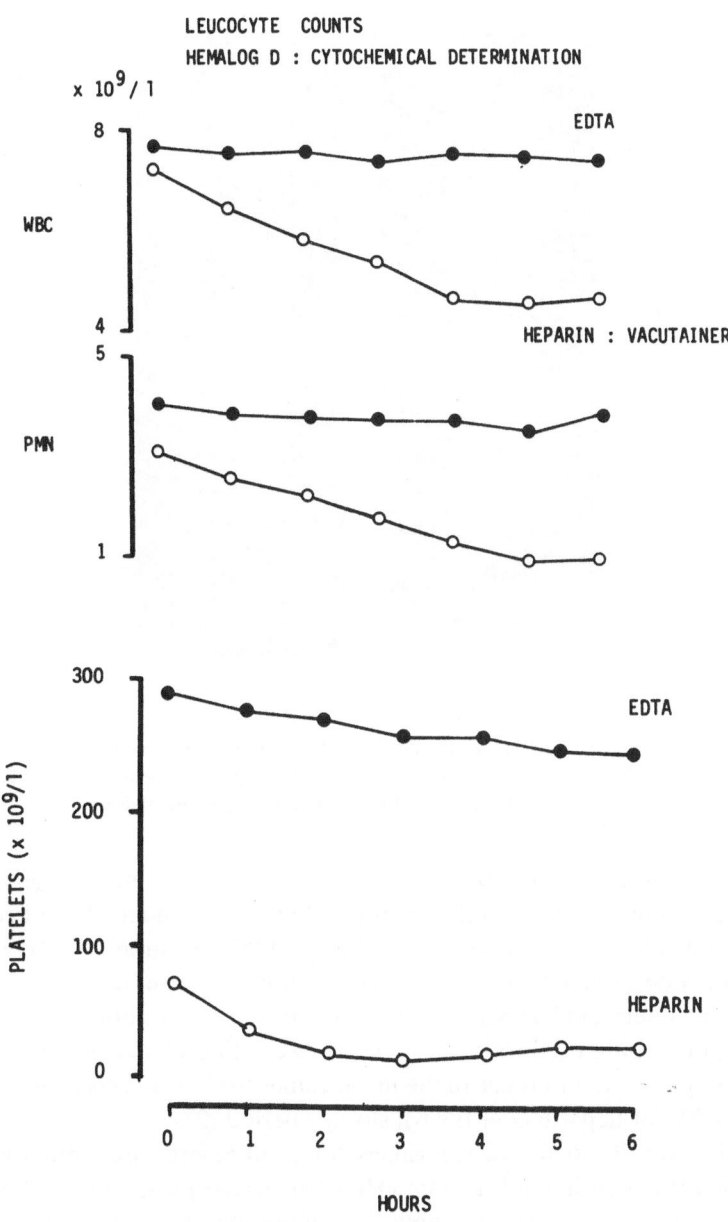

Fig. 2. Effect of storage of whole blood for up to 6 hours on total leucocyte, absolute neutrophil, and platelet counts ($\times 10^9$/l). Mean values for 10 blood samples stored at room temperature.

32

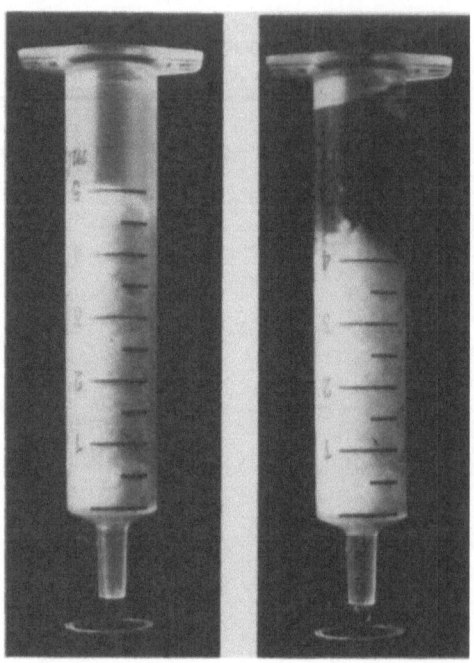

Fig. 3. Plastic syringe containing 1 g of Imugard IG500 cotton wool initially soaked with buffer alone and then with 2 ml anticoagulated blood added to the top of the column. Effluent collected under gravity and washed with buffer prior to testing erythrocyte filterability.

lants on *erythrocyte* filterability are to be studied. Six hour storage experiments, as above, were therefore repeated but, at each hour, the anticoagulated whole blood was passed through Imugard IG500 cotton wool (Fig. 3) as previously described (5, 6). A Neubauer counting chamber was used to check that all platelets and leucocytes had been removed by the cotton wool. When the resulting pure erythrocyte suspensions were filtered at each hour, there was no significant difference in the mean values for P_i for 12 specimens taken into EDTA or heparin over the 6 h storage period (2).

Similar results to the above values for positive-pressure filtration were obtained using an initial-flow-rate (Hémorhéomètre) system (2). The latter instrument was also used to show that defibrinated blood gave the same filtration results as EDTA- and heparin-anticoagulated blood at both 0.5 h and 6 h after venepuncture (2). Thus, provided a pure erythrocyte suspension is studied, there would not seem to be a discernible effect of EDTA or heparin (for up to 6 h at room temperature) on the bulk filtration of normal erythrocytes.

We feel it is important that authors state the source and concentration of anticoagulant used in rheological studies owing to the heterogeneity of commercial anticoagulants, particularly heparin. Although the anticoagulant tubes used in our studies apparently contained a similar stated concentration of heparin per ml of added blood (Sterilin 15 IU/ml; Vacutainer 14.3 USP units ml), chromogenic substrate assays of the plasma heparin concentration, after 1 hour's storage of whole blood at room temperature, gave values 10 times higher for Vacutainer compared with Sterilin tubes (2). The adverse effects of heparin on leucocyte filterability were also found to be correspondingly greater for Vacutainer heparin.

The conclusions of this study apply only to positive-pressure and initial-flow-rate bulk filtration systems and to the commercial forms of anticoagulant we have studied. They do not necessarily apply to other anticoagulant formulations or to more sensitive methods of measuring erythrocyte deformability which, in the future, may be able to demonstrate an anticoagulant effect.

References

1. Stuart, J. and Juhan-Vague, I. (1983). Consideration of the ideal sampling technique, anticoagulant, storage conditions and temperature of measurement. In: Red Cell Deformability and Filterability (Ed. J. Dormandy). Boston, Martinus Nijhoff, pp. 7–15.
2. Lucas, G.S., Caldwell, N.M., Kenny, M.W., Meakin, M., Aillaud, M.F., Billerey, M., Juhan-Vague, I. and Stuart, J. (1984). Effect of calcium-chelating and non-chelating anticoagulants on erythrocyte and leucocyte filterability. Clinical Hemorheology, in press.
3. Stuart, J., Lucas, G.S., Caldwell, N.M., Kenny, M.W., Meakin, M., Aillaud, M.F. and Juhan-Vague, I. (1984). Anticoagulants and erythrocyte filterability. Biorheology, in press.
4. Schröer, R. and Muth, K. (1981). Filtrability of whole blood and erythrocyte suspensions under the influence of several anticoagulants. Ricerca in Clinica e in Laboratorio, *11* (Suppl. 1), 109–116.
5. Kenny, M.W., Meakin, M. and Stuart, J. (1983). Methods for removal of leucocytes and platelets prior to study of erythrocyte deformability. Clinical Hemorheology, *3*, 191–200.
6. Stuart, J., Kenny, M.W., Meakin, M., Lucas, G.S. and Caldwell, N.M. (1984). Leucocyte removal prior to study of erythrocyte deformability. Biorheology, in press.

Effect of time delay from venepuncture on red cell rheology

A.J. Barnes

The effect of storage of blood at room temperature on the measurement of erythrocyte rheology was assessed in 12 normal subjects. Red cell rheology was measured by filtration of whole blood (1), by a micropipette aspiration method (2), by centrifugal packing (3), and by viscometry of packed red cells (4). Measurements were made at 0.5–1.5 h after venepuncture, and again at 24 h, using blood anticoagulated with 1.5 mg/ml K_2EDTA (Seward Laboratory, London). A significant impairment in rheology was observed with the filtration (P<0.01) and micropipette (P<0.02) methods at 24 h but not with centrifugation or packed cell viscometry (Table 1). More detailed studies, where measurements were made at hourly intervals, showed that filtration began to deteriorate at 3 h in some individuals while others did not show changes until 8 h. Using the micropipette method, the earliest changes were detected at 6–8 h from venepuncture. Several variables having a possible effect on erythrocyte deformability were measured within 0.5–1.5 h of venepuncture and at 24 h and are shown in Table 1. It is concluded that following a temperature equilibration period of 0.5 h, blood anticoagulated in K_2EDTA may be

Table 1. Effect of blood storage for 24 h in K_2EDTA – mean (SEM) for 12 normal samples

	0.5–1.5 h	p*	24 h
Mean cell volume (fl)	86.5 (0.3)	<0.02	88.0 (0.6)
Packed cell volume (%)	42.6 (0.8)	<0.02	43.3 (0.7)
Whole-blood filtration (ml/min)	1.38 (0.06)	<0.01	0.48 (0.05)
Micropipette aspiration (mmHg)	1.23 (0.28)	<0.02	1.41 (0.31)
Centrifugal packing (FI 45%)	22.8 (2.0)	NS	20.1 (1.2
Packed red cell viscometry (TK)	0.84 (0.01)	NS	0.83 (0.01)
Plasma viscosity (mPa s)	1.16 (0.04)	NS	1.20 (0.04)
Plasma glucose (mmol/l)	5.3 (0.1)	<0.01	1.8 (0.2)
Plasma sodium (mmol/l)	154 (1.2)	<0.01	158 (1.0)
Plasma potassium (mmol/l)	3.9 (0.2)	<0.02	4.5 (0.2)
Blood pH	7.27 (0.02)	NS	7.24 (0.04)

* Determined by Student's paired t test.

stored at room temperature for 2 h prior to measurement of red cell rheology using the above methods.

References

1. Reid, H.L., Barnes, A.J., Lock, P.J., Dormandy, J.A. and Dormandy, T.L. (1976). A simple method for measuring erythrocyte deformability. Journal of Clinical Pathology, *29*, 855–858.
2. McMillan, D.E., Utterback, N.G. and La Puma, J. (1978). Reduced erythrocyte deformability in diabetes. Diabetes, *27*, 895–901.
3. Sirs, J.A. (1970). Automatic recording of the rate of packing of erythrocytes in blood by a centrifuge. Physics in Medicine and Biology, *15*, 9–14.
4. Dintenfass, L. (1976). Determination of deformability and/or internal viscosity of the blood cells. In: Rheology of Blood in Diagnostic and Preventive Medicine (Ed. L. Dintenfass). London, Butterworths, p. 335.

Red cell age distribution in blood centrifuged to remove leucocytes

M. Hanss

We are currently using a gentle centrifugation technique to obtain a leucocyte-reduced red cell suspension for filtration studies (1). Although the centrifugation speed is low (600 g; the figure was incorrectly reported as 2000 g in the original paper), we felt it necessary to verify that no selection of red cells according to age resulted from the centrifugation.

Pyruvate kinase (PK) activity, which is related to red cell age (2), was measured using standard kits (Boehringer, Mannheim, West Germany). When red cells were centrifuged at 2000 g for 2 h in tubes of 0.5 cm bore and 8 cm length, the following mean (SD) results for PK activity (U/10^{10} red cells) were obtained for 11 samples:

unseparated		–	1.9 (0.5)
red cell layers	– top	–	2.6 (1.0)
	– middle	–	1.6 (0.3)
	– bottom	–	1.3 (0.2)

The top/bottom ratio of 2.0 for PK activity showed that separation of red cells according to age had occurred under these centrifugation conditions. When the gentle centrifugation technique (600 g for 10 min) was used, however, no significant differences in mean (SD) PK activity (U/10^{10} cells) were found between the top – 1.6 (0.4); middle – 1.7 (0.5); and bottom – 1.6 (0.3) layers.

In conclusion, except for possible platelet or red cell aggregates which sediment to the bottom of the tube, sampling of the middle red cell layer after gentle centrifugation allows the preparation of a highly leucocyte-reduced erythrocyte suspension which has, by and large, the same cell age distribution as that of the original blood suspension.

References

1. Hanss, M. (1983). Erythrocyte filtrability measurement by the initial flow rate method. Biorheology, *20*, 199–211.
2. Sass, M.D., Vorsanger, E. and Spear, P.W. (1964). Enzyme activity as an indicator of red cell age. Clinica Chimica Acta, *10*, 21–26.

Erythrocyte volume stability in selected iso-osmotic buffers

H.J. Meiselman

Many studies of the mechanical, geometric and filtration behaviour of human red blood cells (RBC) involve suspending RBC in media other than auto-logous plasma. There thus arises the question of which buffer system to use. In an attempt to answer this question, three iso-osmotic buffer systems were investigated in order to evaluate RBC volume stability in these media; filtra-tion measurements were not made but the results can be related to presently existing literature reports of cell volume versus filtration behaviour.

Three iso-osmotic (290 ± 2 mmol/kg) and constant pH (7.40 ± 0.02 at $25°$ C) buffer systems were used: Tris (tris-hydroxymethyl amino methane – 5, 10, 20, 40 and 50 mM); phosphate (KH_2PO_4 plus Na_2HPO_4 – 30 mM); HEPES (N-2-hydroxyethyl piperazine-N'-2-ethanesulfonic acid – 20 mM). All reagents were of analytical quality and sodium chloride was added to achieve the iso-osmotic condition. Solution osmolality was determined by freezing-point de-pression. Venous blood was taken from healthy donors, using a plastic syringe and 20 G needle, into heparin (5 IU/ml blood) then washed twice and sus-pended, at 10% haematocrit, in the given medium; for the Tris studies, the 5 mM concentration was used for the two washes. The RBC suspensions were incubated at either room temperature ($21 \pm 1°$ C) or $37°$ C and sampled for RBC volume as a function of time. RBC volume was determined using an Electrozone-Celloscope (Particle-Data Inc., Elmhurst, Ill., USA) equipped with a 76 μm orifice and operating at a 15% rejection level to minimise artefacts associated with non-axial transit of particles through the orifice. The suspending media used for these volume determinations were aliquots of those used for preparing the cell suspensions and were pre-filtered through 0.45 μm pore Millipore membranes (Millipore Co., Bedford, Mass., USA).

Volume–time data for RBC in various Tris buffers are shown in Fig. 1 as plots of relative RBC volume versus incubation time; a relative RBC volume of 1.0 indicates no change from the initial control condition. Note that Tris causes an increase in cell volume which is a function of time, concentration, and temperature. Since the relative accuracy of the volume measuring system is in the order of 1%, significant volume increases occurred at $21°$ C for 5 mM at

3 hours, for 10 mM at 2 or more hours, and for 20 mM and greater at 1 hour and beyond. At 37°C, significant increases were noted for 5 mM at 2 hours and beyond, for 10 mM at 1 hour and beyond, and for 20, 40 and 50 mM at one-half hour and beyond. Preliminary data (not shown) indicate that this swelling is not a function of in vivo cell age, in that density-separated young and old RBC exhibited similar volume changes.

A comparison of RBC stability in Tris, phosphate and HEPES buffers is shown in Table 1; the Tris data are taken from Fig. 1. Unlike Tris, the phosphate buffer caused only minimal volume changes which do not appear to be temperature- or time-dependent. RBC in HEPES are the most stable with a mean relative volume of 1.002 (SD 0.005), a value which does not significantly differ from unity. Note that the swelling effects of Tris appear to be due to a modification of the cell membrane leading to a loss of sodium and potassium, with a preferential release of sodium (see ref. 1 for studies of Tris at concentrations greater than 70 mM).

Erythrocyte volume, and thus the cell surface to volume ratio, is known to be an important determinant of RBC deformability. Studies by Hanss (2) and others have shown that the filtration rate of RBC suspensions is markedly reduced when cell volume is increased using hypotonic media. Of particular interest is the report of Leblond (3) who showed that the RBC filtration rate is 40% less for cells in 10 mM Tris than for the same cells in phosphate-buffered saline of the same osmolality and pH. Although volume data were not reported by Leblond, he does indicate that time delays involved in preparing the cells for filtration may have been the basis for the difference; time, plus the data shown in Fig. 1 and Table 1, suggest that volume alterations may have been the basis for the decreased filtration rate when using Tris.

In overview, the results of this study strongly indicate that the use of Tris as a buffer should be avoided in applications where regulation of cell volume is critical (i.e. RBC filtration). Phosphate causes only minimal volume changes,

Table 1. Relative RBC volume in various buffers

Buffer agent	21°C			37°C		
	Time (h)			Time (h)		
	1	2	3	1	2	3
30 mM Phosphate	0.988	0.983	0.975	0.993	0.988	0.987
20 mM Hepes	1.005	1.004	0.995	1.000	1.002	1.008
20 mM Tris	1.023	1.039	1.047	1.054	1.073	1.085
40 mM Tris	1.046	1.081	1.110	1.160	1.206	1.240

Note: All buffers were 290 mmol/kg, pH = 7.4.

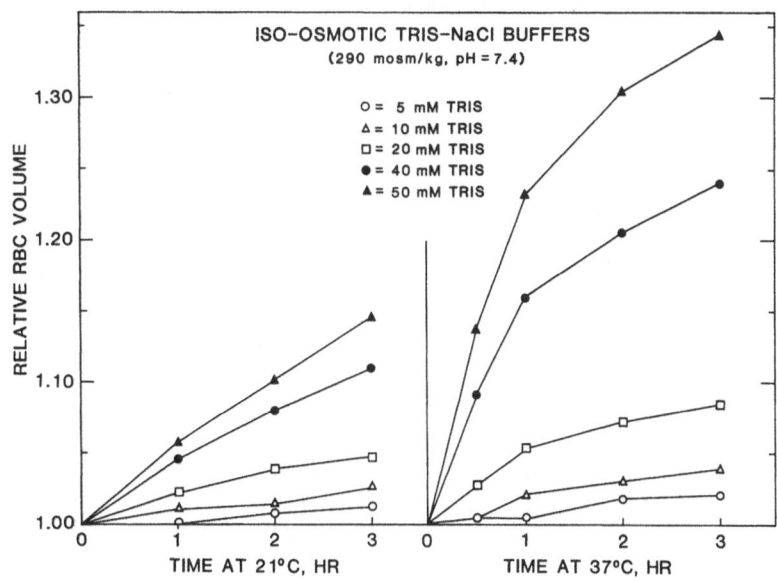

Fig. 1. Volume–time data for RBC suspended in Tris buffer for up to 3 hours at 21 and 37° C.

but does not allow the use of physiological concentrations of metal ions (i.e. calcium) due to the formation of an insoluble precipitate. HEPES, which is one of the 'Good' buffers (4), does not cause any significant change in cell volume for up to 3 hours at 20 mM concentration and, in addition, has the following advantages: (1) it is a zwitterionic buffer and is therefore excluded by biological membranes, (2) its pK is 7.6 and thus close to the normal physiological value, (3) its change of pH with temperature is -0.014 pH units per °C versus -0.31 for Tris, and (4) it does not bind Mg^{2+}, Ca^{2+}, Mn^{2+} or Cu^{2+}. Thus, based solely on volume stability, HEPES appears to be the buffer of choice; additional studies of its effects, if any, on RBC mechanical properties will be needed prior to acceptance of this agent as the ideal 'non-plasma' suspending medium.

References

1. Luthra, M.G., Ekholm, J.E., Kim, H.D. and Hanahan, D.J. (1975). Effects of Tris and histidine on human erythrocytes and conditions influencing their mode of action. Biochimica et Biophysica Acta, *382*, 634–649.
2. Hanss, M. (1983). Plasma and suspending medium. In: Red Cell Deformability and Filterability (Ed. J. Dormandy). Boston, Martinus Nijhoff, pp. 105–107.
3. Leblond, P. (1983). Plasma and suspending medium. In: Red Cell Deformability and Fil-

terability (Ed. J. Dormandy). Boston, Martinus Nijhoff, pp. 108–109.
4. Good, N.E., Winget, G.D., Winter, W., Connolly, T.N., Izawa, S. and Singh, R.M.M. (1966). Hydrogen ion buffers for biological research. Biochemistry, 5, 467–477.

Influence of the suspending medium on red blood cell filtration

S. Coccheri

It is known that the composition of plasma can influence the results of blood cell filtration tests by a direct effect of plasma viscosity on the filtration time and by the effect of plasma proteins on the aggregation of red cells. This concept is especially relevant when testing blood samples from patients with chronic vascular disease, who frequently have quantitatively and/or qualitatively altered fibrinogen, increased α_2-macroglobulin and factor VIII, and raised plasma viscosity. We have therefore studied the influence of different suspension media on red cell filtration in patients with peripheral arterial obliterative disease (PAOD) and intermittent claudication, excluding those with diabetes.

Our filtration method included the following steps:

1. After venepuncture, without stasis, blood was taken into K_2EDTA (final concentration 1.5 mg/ml); leucocytes and platelets were removed by double centrifugation (6 min at 100 g plus 10 min at 2250 g). The residual leucocyte count did not exceed $0.3 \times 10^9/l$.

2. Red cells were then resuspended at 10% (± 0.5) in:

   autologous plasma (AP) – prefiltered through Millipore ($0.22\,\mu m$) filters

   donor plasma (DP) – pooled AB plasma similarly prefiltered

   buffer (B) – Tris-HCl-Ringer-albumin   (pH 7.4) buffer similarly prefiltered

   Red cells had been washed three times with the same suspending medium before final resuspension.

3. Red cell suspensions (1 ml) were filtered through calibrated $5\,\mu m$ pore diameter polycarbonate filters in a Reid-Dormandy type filtration apparatus, under gravity force, at 37° C after 3 min pre-warming.

4. Polycarbonate $5\,\mu m$ pore diameter filters (Nuclepore) were calibrated by twice measuring their filtration time with 1 ml buffer under the same conditions. In the batch of filters used for this study, the mean buffer filtration time (BFT) was 5.9 ± 0.7 s. Only filters with a BFT not exceeding 1 SD (range 5.2–6.6 s) were validated. Filtration of suspen-

sions was performed immediately after calibration.

5. The mean of three measurements was taken as the sample filtration time (SFT). Filtration values were expressed as the ratio between the SFT of suspensions in AP, DP, or B, and the BFT. Our coefficients of variation for these ratios were: 4.9% ± 2.2 for AP; 5.1% ± 2 for DP; 5.3% ± 2.8 for B.

Using this methodology, 11 patients with POAD and 8 control subjects (age and sex matched) have been investigated (Table 1). Although a statistical comparison between POAD patients and controls is premature, it can be seen that only the values for suspensions in autologous plasma (AP) are evidently different in the patients versus the controls. Within the POAD patients, the values for AP were significantly greater (Wilcoxon's rank sum test) than those for B (P<0.02), and greater also than those for DP (P<0.05), although the latter comparison was only at the edge of significance.

From this preliminary study, we can therefore draw the following working hypotheses: (1) prolonged red blood cell filtration times observed in POAD patients may often be the result of the influence of an altered plasma composition (see also ref. 1), and (2) the place of AB donor plasma as a suspending medium for red blood cell filtration should be carefully evaluated, as it may supply a standardised and physiological environment for erythrocytes before and during filtration.

Table 1. Median (range) SFT/BFT ratios of red cell suspensions in different media for 11 patient with POAD and 8 controls.

	Autologous plasma (AP)	Donor plasma (DP)	Buffer (B)
POAD	3.47 (2.48–4.71)	2.98 (2.61–3.54)	2.63 (2.12–3.64)
Controls	2.85 (2.37–4.25)	2.72 (2.41–3.42)	2.60 (2.20–3.33)

Reference

1. Winkenwerder, W., Adams, K., Lineberger, T. and Johnson, G. (1982). Blood filtration in patients with peripheral vascular disease. Clinical Hemorheology, 2, 201–207.

Summary

J. Stuart

It is clear from these studies that the methods used for sample preparation prior to the measurement of erythrocyte deformability are of crucial importance. Since bulk erythrocyte filtration methods are sensitive to the effects of contaminating platelets, leucocytes and plasma proteins, it is essential to remove these extrinsic factors so that a pure erythrocyte suspension can be tested. This can be achieved either by passage of whole blood through cotton wool or by centrifugation at 600 g and aspiration of the middle of the packed erythrocyte layer. Provided one or other of these procedures is used, and the resulting cell suspension is checked visually in a counting chamber, whole blood can be stored for several hours in heparin or K_2EDTA at room temperature prior to testing. Storage for 24 hours or more in citrate-phosphate-dextrose-adenine (blood bank anticoagulant preservative solution) was suggested by Holger Schmid-Schönbein, in discussion, as a possibility for the future. Once resuspended in buffer, the test erythrocytes should be filtered immediately or, if there is any delay, they should not be suspended in Tris buffer since cell swelling will occur. HEPES and phosphate buffers are preferable. An alternative is to resuspend the erythrocytes in standardised donor plasma.

The temperature at which erythrocyte filterability should be tested was also discussed during this session. There was general agreement that temperature-controlled filtration systems should be developed and that a standardised test temperature should be adopted for all laboratories. The recommended temperature should be higher than the anticipated maximum laboratory temperature to avoid the expense of cooling equipment. It was felt that a working temperature of 37° C had obvious advantages provided this could be maintained continuously from the time of removal of the test sample from a water bath until the completion of filtration. This requirement would, however, pose design problems for instrument manufacturers.

During the past year, improvements in erythrocyte filtration methodology have been given priority by the participants in this session. The papers presented reflect the importance of, and continuing need for, collaborative work of this type so that a sound methodological basis can be provided for future clinical studies in haemorheology.

Comparison of different filtration techniques

Summary by G.A. Marcel

I started the session trying to introduce some sort of a regression equation between white cell concentration and various results of filtration indexes analysing both the slope and the intercept of this equation in the hope of being able to distinguish in these experiments what is due to white cells and what is not due to white cells (Fig. 1). I think there is a lot of interpretation to be given to that yet. I also said a few words of changing osmolality by using either sodium chloride or sucrose and differences were shown in the hyperosmolar path (Fig. 2).

John Stuart compared the initial-flow-rate (Hémorhéomètre) method with a modified version of the Birmingham positive-pressure filtration system using the same batch of $5\,\mu$m pore diameter polycarbonate membranes (Nuclepore).

The first important finding was the considerably greater precision that could be obtained with the Hémorhéomètre. A coefficient of variation (CV) of 4.3% for the index of filtration was obtained for 12 separate leucocyte-free suspensions of erythrocytes prepared from one normal blood. The comparable values for 12 erythrocyte suspensions studied by positive-pressure filtration were 10.7% for the initial pressure reading (slope of curve extrapolated back to zero time) and 12.1% for the final pressure (after 5 minutes' filtration). Thus the poorer precision of the Birmingham positive-pressure system should limit its sensitivity, compared with the Hémorhéomètre, to detecting small changes in erythrocyte deformability.

In practice, J. Stuart found that, despite its poorer precision, the positive-pressure system was more sensitive to an in vitro induced loss of erythrocyte deformability. Normal erythrocytes were damaged by heating to 49–50° C for 20 minutes (Fig. 3), by fixation for 60 minutes in varying concentrations of glutaraldehyde (Fig. 4), by oxidative stress to form intracellular Heinz bodies (Fig. 5), and by storing at 4° C for up to 5 weeks in SAGM (sodium chloride, adenine, glucose, mannitol) preservative medium for blood transfusion (Fig. 6). For each of these models he measured the initial pressure and final pressure in the positive-pressure system in comparison with the Hémorhéomètre index

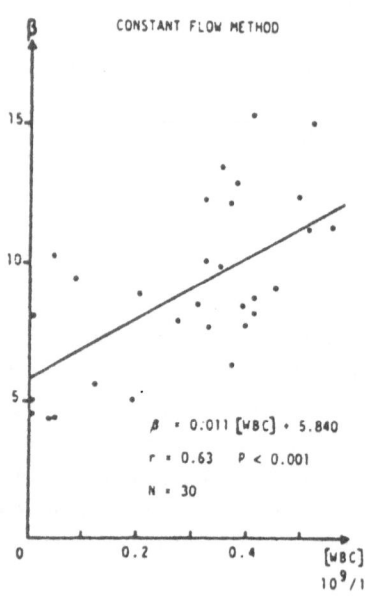

Fig. 1. Variation of β as a funtion of leucocytes.

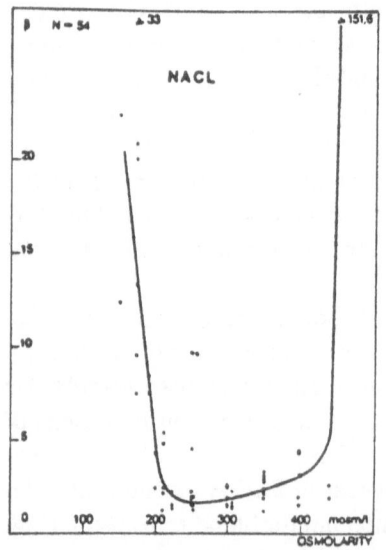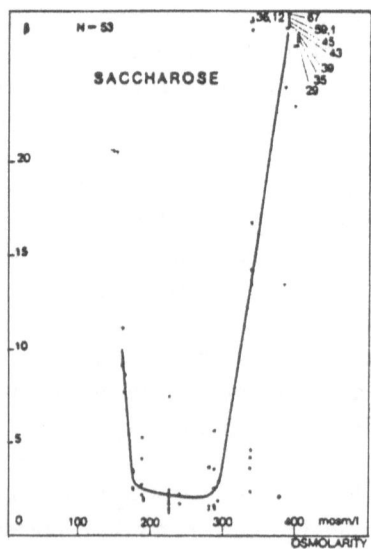

Fig. 2. Variation of β as a function of osmolarity.

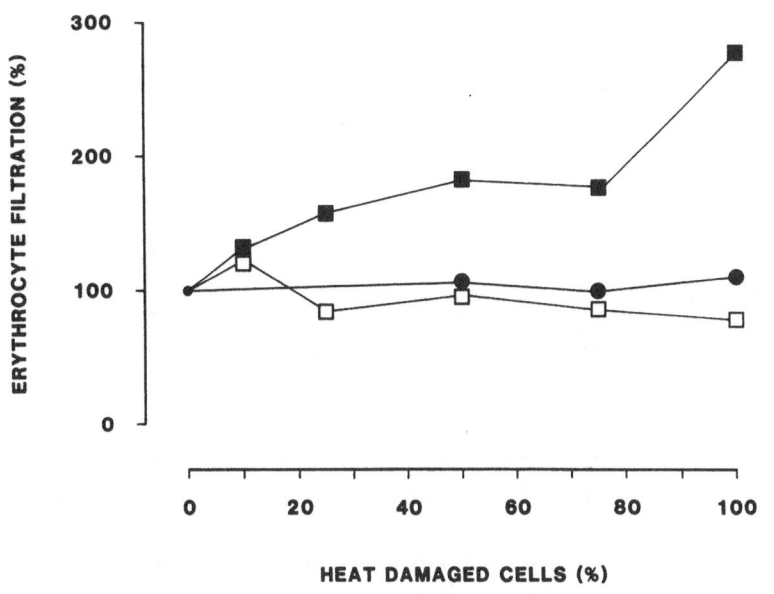

Fig. 3. Effect of an increasing percentage of heat-damaged erythrocytes causing impairment of erythrocyte filtration compared with an initial value expressed as 100% (■ – final positive-pressure, □ – initial positive-pressure, ● – index of filtration).

of filtration. In all four in vitro models, final pressure showed the greatest percentage increase (loss of filterability) as erythrocyte deformability decreased, the first reading being expressed as 100%. Measurement of the index of filtration, again expressed as percentage change, showed the smallest percentage increase (loss of filterability) as erythrocyte deformability decreased. Values for initial pressure tended to be intermediate.

Thus, the Hémorhéomètre index of filtration was surprisingly insensitive to these in vitro test models using artificially-hardened erythrocytes. Further comparisons, using clinical samples as well as in vitro tests, are indicated, but such comparisons should be performed using a positive-pressure filtration system capable of comparable precision with that of the Hémorhéomètre.

Paul Teitel gave us a very detailed talk on the quality of filters and the manners of overcoming this central problem with which we are alle concerned. It is evident that to be used in measurements filters need to be homogeneous, which is not the case with the Nuclepore filters. He devised a method of measuring pneumatic resistivity of each filter. But it is difficult to differentiate results between few pores of great dimensions and many pores with small diameters. The first possibility is to improve the filters – that has been promised for tomorrow. The second possibility is to increase the signal to noise

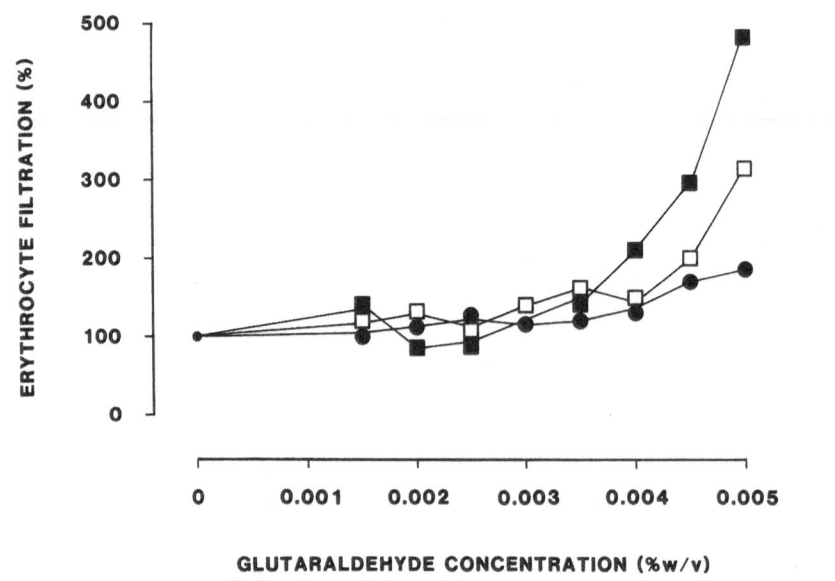

Fig. 4. Effect of incubation for 1 hour in increasing concentrations of glutaraldehyde causing impairment of erythrocyte filtration compared with an initial value expressed as 100% (symbols as Fig. 1).

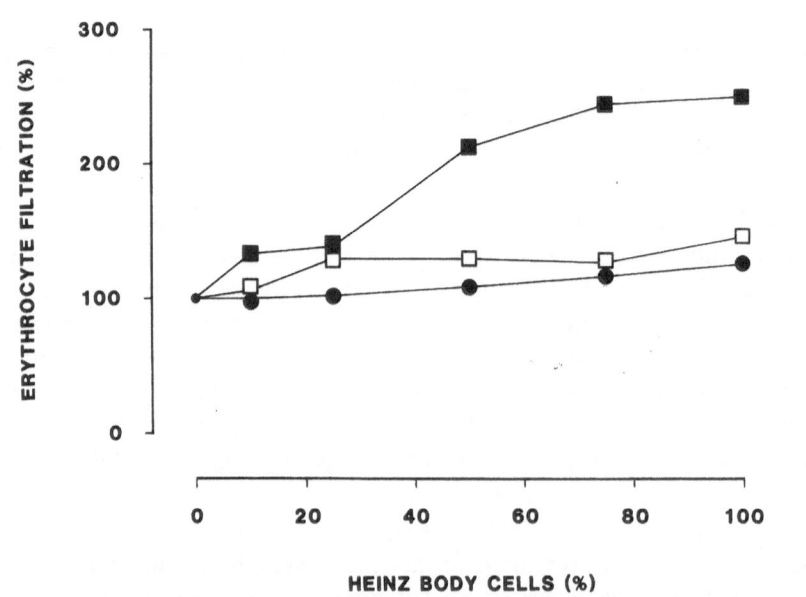

Fig. 5. Effect of an increasing percentage of Heinz body-containing cells causing impairment of erythrocyte filtration compared with an initial value expressed as 100% (symbols as Fig. 1).

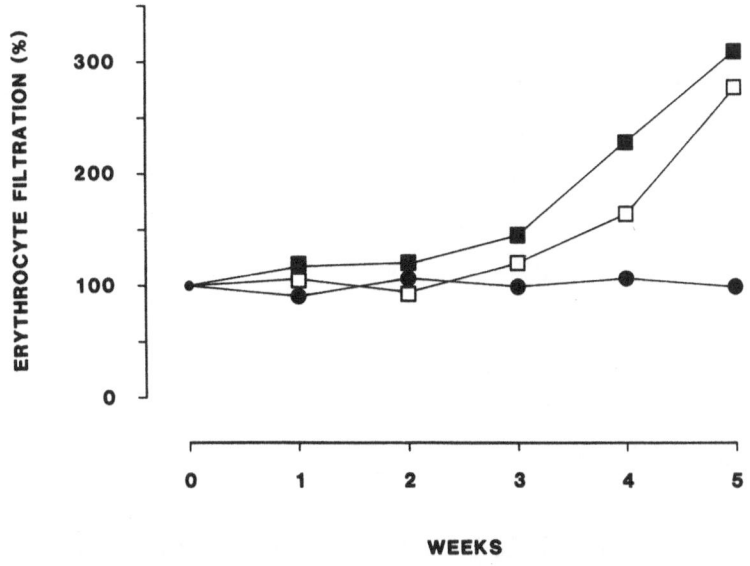

Fig. 6. Effect of storage for 5 weeks in SAGM blood bank preservative solution causing an impairment of erythrocyte filtration compared with an initial value expressed as 100% (symbols as Fig. 1).

ratio by statistical treatment of the data, and this is what was presented, the same elements being measured 12 times with 12 different membranes to pick out the inhomogeneity of the filters. Initial flow rates were plotted against pneumatic resistance and iteration of measurements allows to interpolate results to an acceptable reduction of variation coefficient.

And then we came back to patients with John Dormandy and the work done with Matrai comparing the Reid/Dormandy method, the Dodds modification with lower pressure and haematocrit and buffy coat removed, the Matrai/Dormandy method which was shown to us a bit earlier with lower pressure, 5% haematocrit measuring initial filtration rate and the Hanss method. The author proposed that the most sensitive method to patients was the Hanss method, then came the Matrai/Dormandy method and immediately after and at a similar level the Dodds modification and the original Reid/Dormandy method. This was comparing 11 healthy volunteers to 15 patients with severe ischaemia.

Finally, Michel Boisseau once again gave us arguments for the Hanss method. The first point was comparing erythrocyte sedimentation rate with Reid/Dormandy data and with the Hanss method (Fig. 7). Although it was said that Hanss always found a good correlation between Reid/Dormandy results and erythrocyte sedimentation rate, he discussed this as being due to

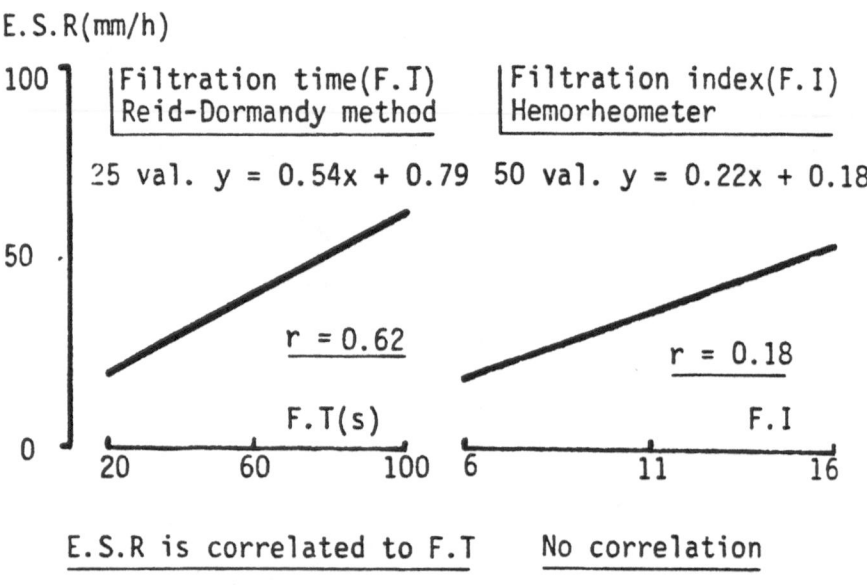

E.S.R(mm/h)

| Filtration time(F.T) | Filtration index(F.I) |
| Reid-Dormandy method | Hemorheometer |

25 val. y = 0.54x + 0.79   50 val. y = 0.22x + 0.18

r = 0.62   r = 0.18

F.T(s)   F.I

E.S.R is correlated to F.T   No correlation

Fig. 7. Erythrocyte sedimentation rate (ESR) and filtration.

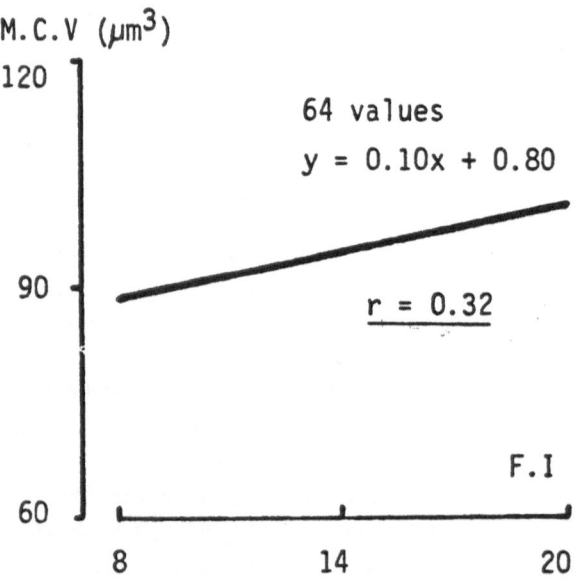

M.C.V (μm^3)

64 values

y = 0.10x + 0.80

r = 0.32

F.I

Fig. 8. Influence of erythrocyte parameter on filtration index (Hémorhéomètre).

fibrinogen or to Factor VIII antigen, and he found no correlation between sedimentation rate and the Hanss method, which of course is a good point for this last method. Then he discussed the comparisons between mean cell volume and the Hanss index (Fig. 8). He found a correlation.

If I may comment on this last session, which was supposed to compare various methods, I feel it would be premature to conclude that there is one single good universal method to be given to all. Not only do we still have a lot of work to do, we should insist, when people ask which method they should use, that they should use a few methods because there are at least two very important fields and methods – the constant pressure methods and the constant flow methods – and we have not quite clarified which is best to use today.

Comparison of blood filtration systems with other techniques for assessing red cell deformability

Introduction

Over the past few years, this Group has accomplished a great deal in clarifying and standardizing the technique of erythrocyte filtration from its numerous original versions. No doubt, the diffusion of this information has already resulted in the publication of more comparable results to the benefit of all those interested in the role played by red cell deformability in various diseases. Yet, aside from filtration, there are several other potentially useful methods that can and have been utilized for the measurement of red cell rheological properties. However, a brief review of the literature indicates that the results obtained by such methods do not always correlate with those obtained by red cell filtration.

   The purpose of this session was precisely to examine the possible causes of such discrepancies and to explore the usefulness of combining and comparing other methods with standard red cell filtration to better understand the role played by the various determinants of erythrocyte deformability in different situations. Six speakers have addressed this question, each in their own way, and I have attempted in the following few pages to summarize their individual contributions, hoping that our mutual friendship will serve as an appropriate buffer to compensate for my partial rendering and possible misunderstanding of their message.

Comparison of red blood cell geometric and viscoelastic properties with various assays of red blood cell deformability: A preliminary analysis

H.J. Meiselman

Professor Meiselman has reviewed and analysed the literature, including some of his own work, on the rheological properties of age-separated adult and neonatal red blood cells studied by three different methods: micropipette aspiration, rheoscopy and filtration.

Adult erythrocytes have been examined from various points of view by several authors. Their so-called 'static' deformability, i.e. that exhibited by cells tested in their resting state (micropipette measurements of SA/V ratio, minimum cylindrical diameter or membrane elastic modulus) does not seem to differ between cells of younger and older age. However, when submitted to dynamic measurements such as in the rheoscope, age-separated subpopulations of red blood cells from adult individuals appear to behave quite differently. As shown in Fig. 1, younger cells deform more easily than older ones at low shear stresses, this difference becoming less and less apparent as the shear stress is increased. Such difference disappears completely when the viscosity of the extracellular medium is increased or when the young cells are osmotically shrunken to the same MCHC and internal viscosity as that of old cells. In other words, older adult erythrocytes deform more slowly than young cells at a given shear stress due to a higher intracytoplasmic viscosity, a rheological feature that cannot be detected by the use of static measurements only. The results of Tillman et al. using a 5 micron pore filtration technique and showing a 25% decrease in the flow rate of old versus young red cells are more difficult to interpret. While this may again reflect a difference in the dynamic deformability of each cell type, Professor Meiselman suggests that this observation may also be explained by the fact that age-separated erythrocytes have different volumes, which results in different numbers of cells per unit of suspension hematocrit and hence different flow rates. The appropriate use of a compensating factor, such as recently suggested by Chien and Skalak ('beta'), may well in this case have resulted in nearly identical flow rates for young and old red cells.

Neonatal erythrocytes, when compared geometrically to unfractionated adult red cells, show a larger diameter, volume and surface area, a 5% smaller

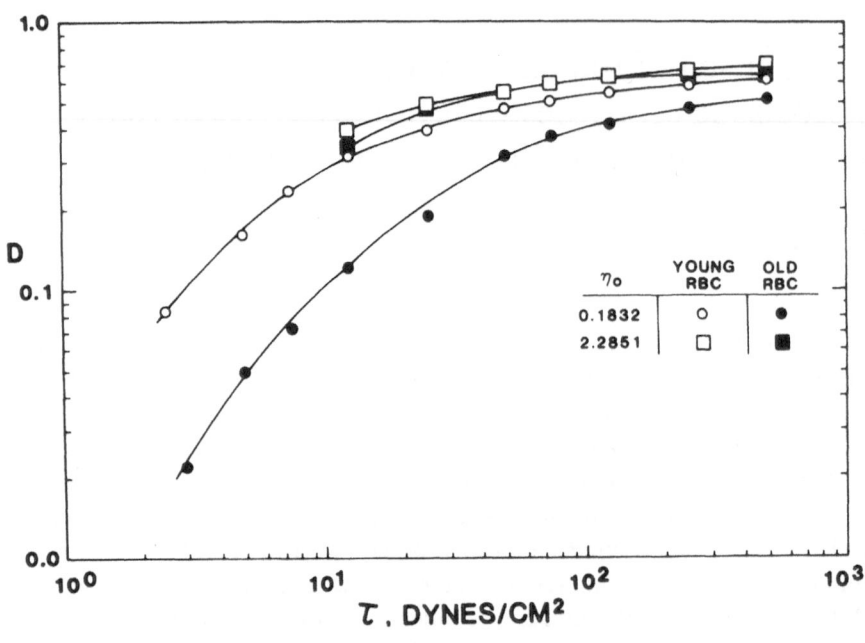

Fig. 1.

Table 1. Adult (A) vs. neonatal (N) filtration (unfractionated RBC).

Study	Suspension	Pores	ΔP	τ, Dynes/ cm^2	Temp.	Findings
Gross and Hathaway, Pediat. Res., 1972	10% HCT in Eagles buffer	$3\,\mu m$	6 cm Hg	5000	25° C	$\dot{Q}_N \approx 0.5\,\dot{Q}_A$ ∴ sign. ↓ for N
Bergquist et al., Bibli. Anat., 1977	2% HCT in saline (hyper, iso, hypo)	$3\,\mu m$ or $8\,\mu m$	15 cm H$_2$O or 25 cm Hg	900 + 2500 or 21,000 + 55,000	23°C	$\dot{Q}_N = \dot{Q}_A$ for all τ and all osmotic conditions
Buchan, Br. J. Haem., 1980	10–15% HCT in plasma	$5\,\mu m$	20 cm H$_2$O	2000	31° C	$\dot{Q}_N = \dot{Q}_A$ but if corrected for plasma N, $\dot{Q}_N \approx 0.9\,\dot{Q}_A$ ($\approx 10\%$ less for N)
Tillman et al., Bibl. Anat., 1981	10% HCT in plasma	$5\,\mu m$	5 cm H$_2$O	500	31° C	$\dot{Q}_N \approx 0.67\,\dot{Q}_A$ ∴ sign. ↓ for N

SA/V ratio and an identical MCHC. Given these geometric properties, it is assumed that methods that are mostly sensitive to differences in the static behaviour of the cells should yield different results, whereas dynamic testing should not. In fact, unfractionated neonatal versus adult red blood cells, when tested in his laboratory using the rheoscope, have shown similar deformability. However, once the cells had been age-separated by centrifugation, young neonatal cells appeared much more deformable than their adult counterparts and, conversely, old ones much less deformable than old adult red cells. This indicates that age-related changes in MCHC and internal viscosity are more pronounced in neonatal than in adult erythrocytes, a phenomenon easily demonstrated with the rheoscope and not with the use of micropipettes. With regard to filtration, published results from experiments comparing unfractionated adult and neonatal red cells are in disagreement, two reports showing no difference at all and two others showing a 50% to 80% decrease in the flow rate of neonatal erythrocytes. Attempts to analyse these studies with respect to such variables as hematocrit, pore size and driving force (Table 1) give no clue as to why these discrepancies exist. In order to resolve this issue, Professor Meiselman suggests that new experiments should be performed under controlled conditions and that proper calculation of the previously mentioned 'beta' factor be applied to account for the difference in cell volume between each population.

Flow techniques and other devices for studying the distribution of the mechanical properties of red blood cells

J.C. Healy and P. Rusch

Professor Healy begins by emphasizing the fact that erythrocytes are often considered as an apparently homogeneous cell population since the results of cytological and biochemical studies are commonly being reported in the form of average values. Yet, everyone knows that erythrocytes represent a distributed population of heterogeneous cells in terms of their density, surface area, volume, diameter, ATP content, etc. In studying the rheological properties of red blood cells, such as membrane viscoelasticity internal viscosity, one should therefore attempt as often as possible to obtain information about the distribution of these features rather than be merely content with the use of techniques that can only provide average values.

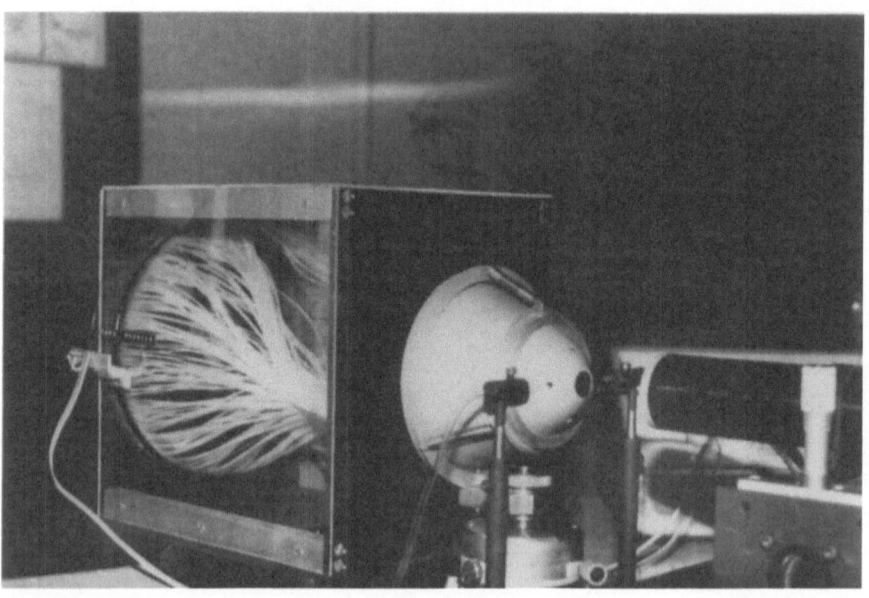

Fig. 1.

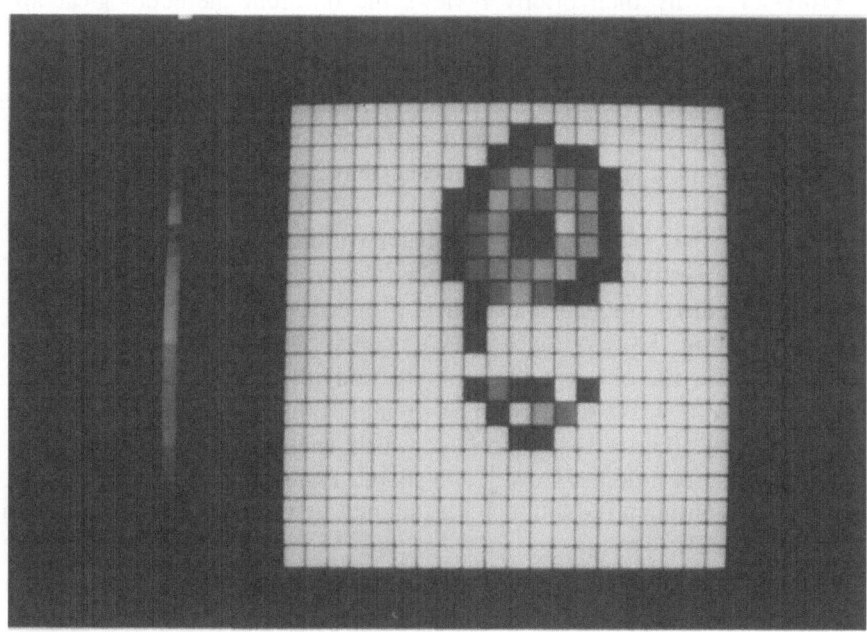

Fig. 2A.

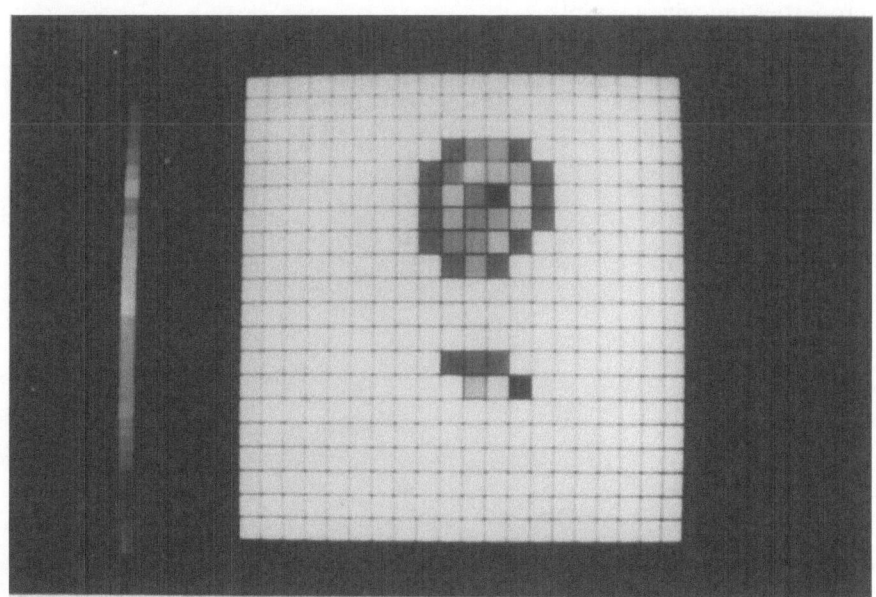

Fig. 2B.

Professor Healy then briefly reviews the different methodological approaches that have been applied to this problem, such as the study of centrifugation-separated subpopulations of erythrocytes with or without the use of sensitizing agents (pH, pO_2, osmolarity), or the application of continuous flow techniques such as the single-pore rigidometer of Kiesewetter which measures the impedance of an electrical current caused by the passage of each individual cell.

Professor Healy and his group have been working recently on the development of a new instrument (Fig. 1) based on the principle of flow-cytometry to examine the distribution of mechanical properties of erythrocytes within a large population. Two approaches have been applied: fluorescence depolarization with the use of a suitable probe to study the intrinsic viscosity of the membrane, and diffractometric measurements taken simultaneously from different angles (between 45° and 145°) which, translated into color intensity diagrams, reflect modifications in cell shape. Figure 2 is an example of the latter, representing a red blood cell examined first at rest (ZA) and then in movement (ZB).

Although this new technology is still in its early stages of development and has not yet been applied to the study of large populations of erythrocytes, Professor Healy concludes that it should be possible soon, by using the vast potential of flow-cytometry and applying it appropriately, to obtain rapid and accurate information about the distributon of individual red cell rheological properties in a given sample.

Comparison of filtration, micropipette aspiration and viscometry in osmotically swollen red blood cells

S. Chien

Osmotic variation in the water content of the red cell is a simple and straight-forward experimental procedure that affects primarily two important determinants of its normal deformability: the SA/V ratio and the intracytoplasmic viscosity. Professor Chien and his colleagues have used this model to test and to compare the sensitivity of three commonly used techniques in their capacity to detect small changes in red cell deformability.

Filtration experiments using Nucleopore membranes were interpreted in terms of the parameter 'beta' which Professor Chien and Professor Skalak have previously shown to describe the average resistance of one cell passing through one pore at a given time. For standard 5 micron pore diameter membranes, they have observed that beta increases very quickly with even a slight decrease in the osmolarity of the suspending medium (250 mosm/l), reflecting the exquisite sensitivity of this method to changes in the SA/V ratio. Within this general description, the comparison of experimental curves obtained with Nucleopore membranes of different pore sizes indicates that filters with smaller pores are relatively more sensitive to geometrical modifications whereas those with larger pores have greater sensitivity to changes in the internal viscosity. This is demonstrated by their observation that the osmolarity value at which the least amount of filtration resistance was observed varies from 350 to 280 to 200 mosm/l for membranes having pore diameters of 3, 5 and 8 microns, respectively.

Micropipettes with small diameter tips (<2 microns) were next utilized to probe the viscoelastic properties of the cell membrane itself. At low osmolarity values, virtually no change was observed from isotonicity, indicating that the method is more sensitive to membrane properties than to overall cell geometry. At osmolarities greater than 400 mosm/l however, they began to observe an increased resistance of the cell to move into the tip of the pipette, reflecting primarily an increase in the viscosity of the membrane itself, probably due to dehydration.

The viscosity of erythrocyte suspensions was finally studied. As expected, this method was particularly sensitive to modifications in the internal viscosity of the cell, especially when the hematocrit of the suspension was adjusted to values of about 80%. Under these circumstances, variations in the osmolarity of the suspending medium resulted in non-linear changes in the apparent viscosity of the entire suspension, reflecting primarily the degree of intracellular hemoglobin concentration.

Professor Chien concludes from these experiments that the three different techniques he has utilized may have quite different sensitivities to the various factors that contribute to the overall deformability of the normal red cell. Such techniques, in his opinion, can be used either alone or in conjunction with one another depending on whether one is interested in a particular aspect only or in a more global assessment of the rheological behaviour of the cell.

Comparison of whole blood filtration with three other methods of assessing red cell rheology in diabetics

A.J. Barnes

Red cell rheology was measured in a group of 100 diabetic patients as part of a study designed to investigate the possible importance of red cell hemorheology on the progression of microcirculatory complications. As there is no generally accepted method for the measurement of cell deformability, this variable was assessed by four previously reported methods in parallel: whole blood filtration (Reid et al.), micropipette aspiration (McMillan et al.), centrifugal packing (Sirs) and packed red cell viscometry (Dintenfass).

Figure 1 demonstrates erythrocyte rheology in diabetics to be impaired as judged from filtration measurement by viscometry (TK) and improved as assessed by centrifugation. No difference is seen in packed cell viscometry. Preliminary micropipette studies suggest a slight increase in flow resistance in

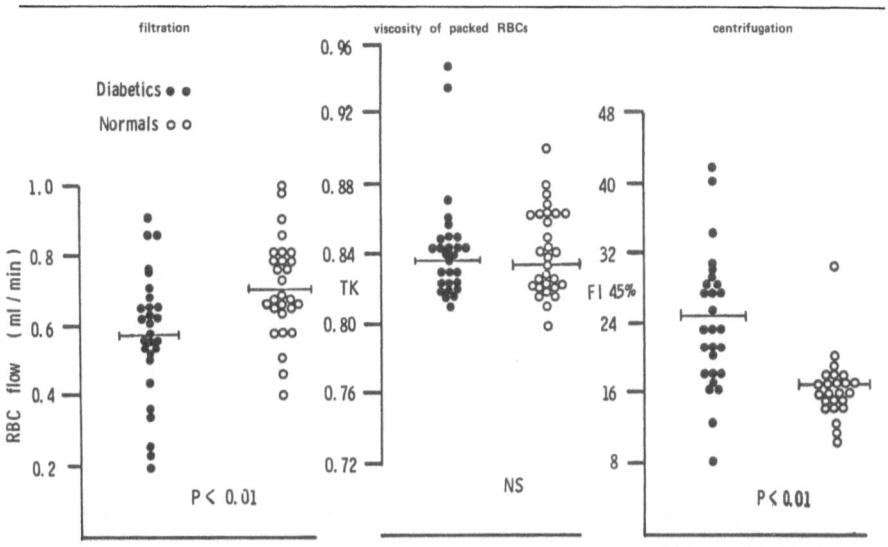

Fig. 1. Red cell rheology measurements in diabetic patients and controls as assessed by three methods.

diabetic red cells in plasma that may be largely due to an increase in plasma viscosity.

Simple bivariate analysis demonstrated a weak positive correlation between whole blood filtration and micropipette red cell flow resistance in plasma ($r = 0.31$, $p < 0.05$). Filtration and erythrocyte flexibility measured by centrifugation were inversely correlated ($r = -0.33$, $p < 0.01$) but again, observations showed a large scatter. Filtration did not correlate with the TK value (packed red cell viscometry).

Professor Barnes concludes that differences in methodology for the measurement of erythrocyte deformability may lead to widely varying results. The method most suitable for the clinical evaluation of patients remains to be determned by prospective long-term studies.

Preliminary report on the use of a new reusable metallic filter membrane

H. Schmid-Schönbein

Professor Schmid-Schönbein reminds the group of the existence of a large coefficient of variation in the results of filtration experiments that have been reported by most authors in the literature. This, he feels, remains a major problem due to the widespread use of disposable polycarbonate membranes having an intrinsic variability in their pore diameter and pore density.

In order to improve on this weak part of the filtration technique, Professor Schmid-Schönbein and his coworkers at Aächen have begun to experiment with the use of a new reusable metallic filter of 12.5 micrometers in thickness having a very uniform pore diameter distribution (3.86 ± 0.34 micrometers) with constant pore density and absence of doublets. A first slide showing the results of hydraulic resistance tests performed during and after repeated use of this membrane shows great reproducibility throughout. The membrane was next tested in Teitel's polymicroviscometer instrument with suspensions of osmotically shrunken red blood cells and the results analyzed with the statistical enhancement method of interpolation described in a previous session of this meeting. The coefficient of variation observed for several experiments performed under these conditions was of the order of only 3%, as compared to 50% or more by Nucleopore filtration techniques.

Professor Schmid-Schönbein concludes that these results represent a considerable improvement owing primarily to the fact that such a membrane, after being carefully calibrated, can be reutilized as often as necessary.

Comparison of different types of filters with the use of erythrocytes with artificially bridged membranes

P. Teitel

In a technique recently described by Thomas Fischer, red cells incubated in hypertonic solutions and then heated at 46° C to partially denaturate their spectrin become firmly attached by a point of membrane contact. When resuspended in isotonic solutions these cells regain their original state of hydration but remain 'bridged' at the dimple in such a manner that they can no longer tanktread. Otherwise, the cells are normally deformable in the sense that their membrane can easily fold into the tip of a small micropipette and that their internal viscosity remains unchanged.

Red blood cells prepared in this manner were tested with different filtration techniques using different types of membranes. In situations of 'restricted pore passage', such as with Nucleopore filters or in the single cell rigidometer, the observed flow rates for suspensions of bridged versus control erythrocytes were virtually the same, indicating that a geometrically restrictive pore system cannot detect the existence of a bridged membrane despite its inability to tanktread. If, on the other hand, one uses the polymicroviscometer which is characterized by the existence of numerous long and branching channels with a non-restrictive diameter, the presence of bridged erythrocytes is clearly detected by a slower and more irregular flow rate than that observed with normal red cells. This confirms the important role of tanktreading in the flow of packed erythrocytes at very low rates of shear. A similar phenomenon can be observed if one uses nucleated avian erythrocytes or even human dehydrated red cells, both of which are unable to tanktread but have been shown previously by Shu Chien to flow easily across restrictive Nucleopore membranes.

Professor Teitel mentions next that in contrast with these bridged-membrane erythrocytes, red cells that have been treated with diamide + iodoacetate in order to specifically crosslink their spectrin are still capable of tanktreading and therefore of flowing quite normally in the polymicroviscometer despite their reduced compliance to shear-elongation when tested for instance in a rheoscope or an ektacytometer. This, he points out, is different from treatment with diamide *alone* which, like NEM, does not protect other membrane sulfhydryl groups and results in a complete rigidification of the membrane that is easily detected with the use of Nucleopore or similar filters.

The conclusion here again is that different methods, when applied to assess the deformability of specifically altered red blood cells, have different sensitivities to the various factors involved. They should therefore be used after careful choice and with proper interpretation of their results.

New evidence on possible clinical relevance of blood filtration systems

Whole blood filtration in diabetes: What is its clinical meaning?

A.J. Barnes

Many cross sectional studies of blood filtration and other rheological variables have now been carried out in diabetic patients. Most of these have shown impaired red cell or whole blood filtration in diabetics which several groups have found to be most striking in those individuals with circulatory and microcirculatory complications. However, these studies provide no indication as to whether diabetic complications are a consequence of altered rheology or whether both might be secondary to some metabolic or other disturbance. Further information on the importance of altered filtration in diabetics might be gained by careful prospective longitudinal studies in which rheological variables are observed in relation to the progression of microcirculatory disease.

A 12-month pilot study was carried out in order to determine the relationship between whole blood filtration and other variables on the progression of diabetic complications. Nine insulin-dependent diabetic patients were transferred from conventional twice daily insulin injections to continuous subcutaneous insulin infusion (CSII) in order to optimise their metabolic control and in this way possibly improve their blood rheology. HbA1C fell from a mean value of 10.7% to 8.7% in this group but there was no change in the levels of this index of metabolic balance in four additional control diabetics who remained on twice daily insulin for 12 months. Over the 12 month period there was a significant improvement in whole blood viscosity and in PCV in the CSII group but there was no change in plasma viscosity and filtration or red cell rheology as measured by filtration or centrifugation. In 5 out of the 9 patients retinopathy showed photographic evidence of progression. Neither the initial levels of rheological or metabolic variables nor their change in response to improved control appeared to predict in which patients retinopathy remained static and in which retinopathy progressed.

As this study was of short duration and the number of patients studied comparatively small, two further prospective investigations have now been initiated:

(a) A 3-year longitudinal study of 100 diabetic patients attending a specialist diabetic retinopathy referral clinic. The power of initial levels of different rheological variables including blood filtration, in predicting the natural history of diabetic retinopathy as quantitated by serial retinal photography will be assessed. Results should be available at the end of 1984.

(b) Seven hundred diabetics at a district general hospital diabetic clinic are currently being screened by whole blood filtration. All patients with filtration values greater than 2 standard deviations above the control mean will be followed longitudinally for 3 years to determine (a) the consistency of their abnormal filtration and (b) the natural history of any complications when compared to patients with normal blood filtration.

Clinical relevance of the Siena technique

F. Laghi Pasini

In our clinical and experimental studies of the rheological properties of blood, we have employed, for several years, the classical Reid-Dormandy technique modified by measuring immediately after venepuncture at 37°C, and with slight anticoagulant excess. Whole blood filterability has been correlated with other rheological parameters such as blood, plasma and serum viscosity, haematocrit and fibrinogen.

Our studies have shown that in chronic coronary artery disease, in acute myocardial infarction and in angina pectoris these is a significant decrease of whole blood filtration rate. These changes seem to be proportional to the severity of the disease, develop rapidly and are reversible in acute spontaneous or provoked ischaemic conditions. Similar findings are observed in claudicants, where red cell filterability is impaired under basal conditions and further decreases during claudication.

Rheological changes have been observed also in other populations of patients suffering from different pathological conditions in which an ischaemic process is not involved. For instance, we have found significant decrease of whole blood filtration rate in untreated hypertensive patients, independently from the severity of the haemodynamic defect.

Finally, our more recent data concern a study on cerebrovascular patients. Cerebral infarction is associated with an increase of whole blood viscosity and decrease of blood filtration rate. In TIA patients such modifications are evident in the acute phase. An increase of fibrinogen concentration is present in cerebral infarction as well as in TIA, while an increase of haematocrit is evident only in TIA patients. There is also an increase of plasma and serum viscosity. However, fibrinogen increase appears rather later and it is apparently unrelated to plasma viscosity curve. Changes in blood viscosity and filtration rate are maximal at the onset of the stroke and progressively return to their basal values, showing a good correlation with clinical evolution. We must emphasise that in TIA patients the changes of filtration rate are as rapid and transient as during angina pectoris. The findings obtained in cerebrovascular patients are in agreement with those obtained in other acute ischaemic conditions. They also confirm that whole blood filterability changes measured by means of our method may have a significant diagnostic and prognostic value. Moreover, we believe filtration rate changes are more evident and more sensible than blood or plasma viscosity changes.

Prognostic significance of whole blood filtration test in patients with cerebral infarction

M.R. Boisseau

Several authors have recently pointed out the relationship between the decrease of blood filterability and prognosis in cerebral infarction. We have analysed this problem in a well-defined group of patients with cerebral infarction using the whole blood filtration technique. Sixteen patients were carefully selected by CAT scan examination, with recent cerebral infarction due to atherosclerosis, without haemorrhage. Blood filterability was measured by the Reid and Dormandy method, weekly during the first three weeks.

Patients with cerebrovascular accidents had a reduced filtration rate compared to control. In the 16 patients the filtration rate in those who survived was 57 ± 24 compared to 34 ± 11 in the subjects who subsequently died. This difference was significant ($p<0.005$). We confirmed therefore that patients with cerebrovascular accidents have a reduced filtration rate during the acute phase. In addition, decreased filterability of the blood carries a bad prognosis. The respective roles of plasmatic and red cell disturbances remain to be determined. It must be pointed out that this phenomenon occurs at the same time as the haemoconcentration is corrected therapeutically, which favours the hypothesis that the decreased filterability is mainly due to a red cell abnormality.

Summary

J.A. Dormandy

Dr Barnes described the turmoil in diabetic circles; for instance, none of the rheological measurements were able to predict deterioration in retinopathy over a year. On the other hand we also learned that improvement in all existing classical biochemical changes associated with diabetes does not seem to be accompanied by a clinical improvement, in the preliminary analysis of a large trial. He also reported on a large-scale screening programme that he has started in diabetics using the Reid and Dormandy technique and showed that there was no correlation with the ESR which is contrary to the data presented earlier at this meeting. He said that in relation to diabetes it is impossible to be certain as yet whether impaired filtration is a reproducible entity, whether it reflects diabetic control, or if it predicts the onset or progression of complications. Although Dr Barnes had used various techniques for assessing red cell filterability, he chose a single filtration technique for his large-scale diabetic screening programme because it was the simplest.

Dr Juhan showed us that abnormalities in the lipid composition of the red cell membrane are related to the fluidity of the membrane, and she tried to relate this to the changes in blood filterability which she had demonstrated in diabetics. On an artificial pancreas the cholesterol/phospholipid ratio was improved within a matter of hours, and this may be related to the parallel changes in blood filterability.

When I tried to resurrect the Reid technique, Dr Lowe commented that in epidemiological studies the haematocrit, fibrinogen and the white cell counts were the best predictors of cardiovascular disease. These three – the haematocrit, fibrinogen and the white cell count – are also the most important determinants of the results obtained with the Reid technique. Professor Schmid-Schönbein put the case against using this technique because it measured too many factors and it was an impure test.

Dr Laghi Pasini presented results from Siena using a modified Reid method. He reminded us that ischaemia, both chronic and acute, in the myocardial, cerebral and leg circulation was associated with a very marked decrease in filterability. The onset could be over a period of minutes and the changes were rapidly reversible. Professor Stuart believed that these acute changes could be explained on the basis of acute phase reactants, while Dr Lowe and I thought that although acute phase reactants obviously do play a part they could not explain all the changes in filterability that occur so rapidly.

Professor Boisseau presented his data on cerebrovascular accidents, again using the Reid technique. He pointed out that febrile patients had a lower filterability and that this was not due to an increase in the white cell count. He also showed us data that red cell filterability after ischaemic cerebral attacks was a good predictor of survival or death within the subsequent 30 days.

Professor Coccheri made several interesting points and drew our attention to the importance of defining the aims and objectives of filtration tests. He suggested the possible value of a test which could pick out those who were at greatest risk in the future from an apparently healthy normal population.

The best feasible protocol for investigating the clinical effect of a haemorheological agent in leg ischaemia

S. Chien, J.A. Dormandy and R. Skalak

1. Aim of study

Primary aim

To assess whether a haemorheologically active agent given long-term orally has a beneficial clinical effect in patients with intermittent claudication.

Secondary aim

Is there a correlation between the clinical course of patients (treated and untreated) and particular haemorheological measurements?

2. Design

Multicentre
Double-blind
Randomised with a placebo
Placebo run-in

3. Patient selection

3.1 Patients with classical intermittent claudication due to atherosclerotic disease, without rest pain or gangrene.

3.2 *Exclusion criteria*

1. One palpable arterial pulse in both feet.
2. Doppler pressure index above 0.85 in both feet.
3. Symptoms or signs suggesting possible neurological claudication.
4. Clinical or laboratory evidence of a classical primary haemorheological disease, such as myelomatosis or leukaemia.
5. Gangrene or ulceration of either foot.
6. Onset of symptoms within past three months.
7. Acute deterioration of symptoms within past one month.
8. Arterial reconstruction or sympathectomy within one month.
9. Patients taking other drugs with possible haemorheological effect during past month.
10. Patients clinically unstable during placebo run-in period (see 4.3.5).

11. Patients where consistent haemorheological and laboratory data cannot be obtained in either the run-in or in the last month of treatment (see 4.3.5).

3.3 *Notes on exclusion criteria*

1. Criteria 1 to 4 are designed to exclude patients who may not have classical arterial intermittent claudication.
2. Criteria 5 is designed to exclude 'end-stage' disease. Fontaine classification IV.
3. Criteria 6 to 8 are designed to exclude patients whose natural history is likely to be unstable.
4. Note that there is no exclusion on the basis of age, sex or other co-existing disease such as diabetes.
5. Criteria 10 and 11 are designed to exclude patients where reliable objective data cannot be obtained.

4. Number of centres, patients and estimated duration of trial

Maximum number of five centres.

Minimum number of patients entering trial after completing run-in period: 1 per week per centre.

(With, say, 4 centres, a minimum of 100 patients will enter trial in six months.)

Aiming to finish with at least 100 completed results, entry into the trial should continue until 130 patients are on the actual double-blind phase.

Including an initial period of standardisation of measurement techniques, the whole trial should be completed well within 2 years.

5 Study plan

5.1 *General principles*

1. All patients seen at least once a month throughout the study of minimise drop-out rate.
2. Each patient to be seen by the same doctor on each visit; again to maintain their continuing co-operation.
3. Standardisation of patient selection, entry criteria, heamodynamic measurements and general data quality.
4. Standardisation and quality control of laboratory measurements.
5. A placebo run-in period to eliminate variable placebo response and ensure a stable initial baseline, both clinically and in terms of physiological haemodynamic measurements.
6. Exclusion of patients where consistent objective data cannot be obtained during last month of treatment (see 6.2 below).
7. No stratification.

80

5.2 *Run-in period on placebo* (see trial schema 5.4)

All patients fulfilling entry criteria will be given placebo for two months with full set of physiological measurements at 0, 1 and 2 months. If 'objective' physiological measurement at 1 and 2 months differs by more than the change specified below, they will be excluded from the trial proper:

Step Test. Time to beginning of claudication	20% change
Step Test. Maximum time possible	20% change
Pacemeter reading over two weeks	20% change
Resting ankle/arm pressure ratio in worse leg	10% change
Post ischaemia/arm pressure ratio in worse leg	10% change
Post ischaemia peak calf blood flow in worse leg	15%

Time to post ischaemia peak calf blood flow in worse leg 15% change (Any greater change in any of these measurements will exclude the patient from the trial proper as specified in exclusion criteria 4.2.10.) Note: Alternatively, the placebo run-in period could be continued until the patient's measurements do stabalise in the rest limits.

5.3 *Double-blind trial period*

Patients qualifying for entry will be randomly allocated to the test and placebo group. They will continue on that treatment for 1 year with full assessment at 6 months, 11 months and 1 year. They will, however, be seen and assessed clinically every month. Patients whose 'objective' measurements at 11 months and 1 year differ by more than specified in 6.2 above will also be excluded (see criteria 11).

At the end of the year's treatment and assessment, all patients will be given the test substance if they wish. (The code, however, will not be broken until the whole trial is completed.)

Alternatively, a placebo 'run-out' period may be advisable.

5.4 *Trial schema*

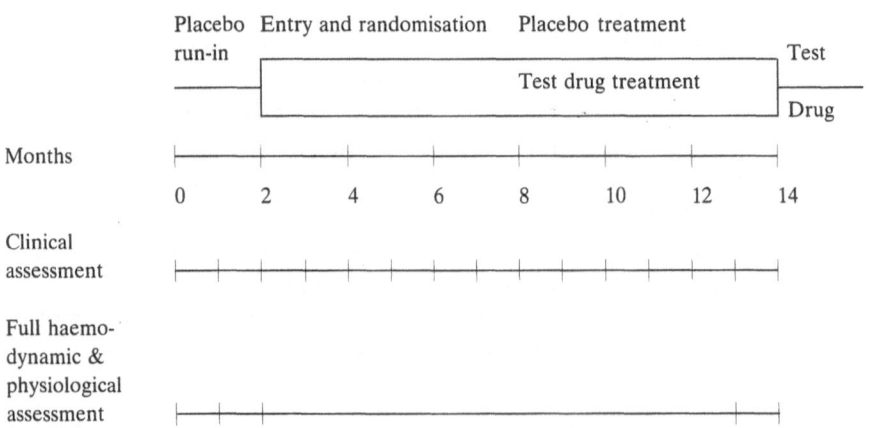

6. Clinical assessment

6.1 *Initial history*

1. General details (age, sex, weight, etc)
2. Onset of claudication (when acute or gradual)
3. Which leg is limiting walking
4. Claudication distance now
5. Change over past month
6. Present medications
7. Previous medication
8. Co-existent disease: Diabetes
   Angina
   Myocardial infarction
   Hypertension
   Cerebral ischaemia
   Others
9. Smoking habits (duration and quantity now)

6.2 *Symptoms*

Change in claudication distance
Change in circumstances of claudication (e.g. patient can now 'walk through' claudication, which he could not before)
Onset of rest pain
Change in work or leisure exercise
Change in means of regular transport (e.g. to and from work)
Other medical events since last visit
Change in medication
Possible side effects
Change in smoking habits

6.3 *Signs*

Full cardiovascular examination including weight, blood pressure, leg pulses, trophic changes etc.

7. 'Objective' physiological/haemodynamic measurements

7.1 *Step Test*

Patient to walk up and down three 9″ (22 cm) steps at the rate of one step per second, timed by a metronome. Time to onset of claudication recorded and patient then encouraged to continue as long as possible. Maximum time recorded.
Note: This is an alternative to the traditional treadmill test which may be more difficult to standarise at several centres

7.2 *Pacemeter (Pedometer)*

Patient provided with a pacemeter and instructed to attach it to his/her waist during waking hours. To be read at two weekly intervals during run-in period and again during last month of trial. Note: Although an unusual technique, it is not only cheap but may be very relevant to patients' symptoms.

7.3 *Doppler systolic pressures at ankle*

Patient to rest horizontally for 15 months before test. Using any type of Doppler flowmeter the systolic pressure is determined in the dorsalis pedis and posterior tibial arteries of both legs. The blood pressure in the right arm is recorded at the same time with a sphygmomanometer.

7.4 *Post ischaemia ankle/arm ratio*

Using the ankle artery with the lowest recordable pressure, the pressures are recorded at 30 second intervals following three minutes of total ischaemia. Total ischaemia is obtained by a wide thigh cuff inflated to suprasystolic pressure. The arm blood pressure is also recorded as soon as possible after the ischaemia.

7.5 *Calf blood flow*

This is measured with any reliable type of venous occlusion plethyamograph, in the worse leg. Readings at rest until steady state is reached. Measurements are repeated as frequently as possible starting immediately after another 3 minute period of total ischaemia. The peak post-ischaemic calf flow as well as the time to reach peak flow are recorded.

7.6. *Additional measurements*

The above measurements (8.1 to 8.5) will be carried out at all centres. Additional measurements aimed at assessing the circulation may be carried out where facilities exist. For instance:

1. Percutaneous pO_2
2. Muscle pO_2
3. Radioactive clearance from muscle
4. Thermography
5. Fluorescein angiography
6. Skin temperature under controlled conditions

8. Laboratory and haemorheological assessment

8.1 *Blood sample*

To be drawn without stasis into EDTA-containing tubes for measurements on red cell suspensions. Centrifuge to separate plasma (for plasma viscosity and protein measurement) and blood cells. The packed cells will be diluted in isotonic buffer and passed through cotton wool to remove WBCs and platelets (preparation of red cell suspensions). Heparin to be used as anticoagulant for measurements on whole blood.

8.2 *Bulk rheological measurements*

8.2.1 *Viscometer:* Rotational or capillary viscometer with controlled

shear rates (high shear rate $\geq 200\,s^{-1}$; low shear rate $0.1-1\,s^{-1}$).
Measurements made at controlled temperature (preferably
$37°\,C$).

8.2.2 *Plasma viscosity:* In rotational viscometers must ascertain the
absence of surface layers, which can be prevented with a guard
ring.

8.2.3 *Blood viscosity:* Viscosity of original whole blood at two or more
shear rates. Sample should be well mixed prior to each measurement (at each shear rate).

8.3 *Filterability measurement*

8.3.1. *Filtration methodology:* Polycarbonate sieves with $5\,\mu$ pores.
Determine pore density and pore diameter distribution before
usage. For constant-pressure (P) technique, the flow rate (Q) is
determined. For constant-flow technique, pressure is determined. The P/Q ratio is the flow resistance (R). Determine R_o
for each filter with the cell-free buffer solution prior to filtration
of suspensions or blood. The wall shear stress in the filter pore
$(= Pr/2l)$ should be kept low (preferably $<100\,dyn/cm^2$)

8.3.2 *Filtration of whole blood*

8.3.3 Filtration of RBC suspensions: the cotton-wool filtered packed
cells will be washed once in a large volume of buffer solution and
then re-suspended in the same buffer at a haematocrit of 10%.

8.3.4 *Filtration of plasma*

8.3.5 *Calculation and expression of results:* for the filtration of whole
blood and RBC suspensions, it is desirable to obtain the resistance–time curve for a period of time (e.g. 1 min). The initial
resistance (R_i) will be determined and expressed as a relative
initial resistance (R_{ri}):

$$R_{ri} = R_i/R_o$$

For the RBC suspension, a rigidity index of a single RBC in a
single pore (R.I.) can be calculated as:

$$R.I. = \frac{(R_{ri} - 1)}{H}\ \frac{V_c}{V_p} + 1$$

where H is the fractional haematocrit, V_c is the mean corpuscu-
lar volume and V_p is the mean pore volume $(= \pi_r^2 l)$.

The later phase of the filtration curve can be usd to estimate the
rate of filter pore plugging (by rigid RBCs or by WBSs).

8.4 *Measurement of RBC aggregation:* by light transmission or light reflec-
tion measurements under controlled shear rates.

8.5. *Haematological measurement on whole blood and RBC suspension:*

    8.5.1 Red cell indices: Haematocrit, red cell count, haemoglobin concentration

    8.5.2 White cell count and differential. Platelet count.

    8.5.3 Plasma protein concentration (total concentration and fractions, fibrinogen).

    8.5.4 Blood cell morphology: by light microscopy on wet suspensions and by scanning electron microscopy.

9. End points

  9.1 All patients who completed one year of treatment and whose 11 and 12 months' objective assessment fall within the limits stated in 6.2 above will be analysed.

  9.2 In addition, patients withdrawn from the trial because of documented deterioration in their circulation to the leg necessitating more active intervention will also be analysed separately. All objective measurements must be repeated before withdrawal. To qualify for analysis, withdrawal from the trial must be for one of the following reasons:

    1. Rest pain, at least once a day for seven consecutive days.

    2. Ischaemic ulcer, which does not heal with usual measures during one month.

    3. Frank gangrene.

    4. Significant deterioration in symptoms or signs of ischaemia requiring surgical intervention.

  9.3 Protocol to be submitted to an expert medical statistician for advice and appropriate modification.

Classified bibliography

G.D.O. Lowe

Aim. List of published/in press papers on relationships of blood filtration to methodology, blood components, and disease states, classified accordingly.
Why? To help the struggling filterer to keep his head above the rising sea of literature. 'He who ignores history is condemned to repeat it'. Note the limited bibliographies in reports of First and Second Workshops.
Scope. Full publications, not abstracts. For brevity, only first author given and title omitted. Conclusions omitted (often not warranted!) Drug effects omitted – recent reviews available (G.A. Marcel, 2nd Workshop Report, pp 214–215; G.D.O. Lowe, Clin. Hemorheol., 1984, in press).

1. Reviews

(a) Previous reports of Working Group
    Lowe, G.D.O. Clin. Hemorheol., 1981, *1*, 513–526. (1st report).
    Dormandy, J.A. (ed.). Red Cell Deformability and Filterability. Boston,
        Martinus Nijhoff, 1983. (2nd report).

(b) Other reviews
    Bessis, M. et al. (eds.). Red Cell Rheology. Blood Cells, *3, Parts 1–2.*
        Berlin, Springer Verlag, 1977. (Paris Symposium).
    Scand. J. Clin. Lab. Invest., 1981, *41, Suppl. 156.* (Goteborg Symposium).
    Chein, S. Blood Cells, 1977, *3*, 71–90.
    Chein, S. Scand. J. Clin. Lab. Invest., 1981, *41, Suppl. 156*, 7–12.
    Weed, R.I. Am. J. Med., 1970, *49*, 147–150.
    Anon., Lancet, 1978, *ii*, 1348–9.
    Rice-Evans, C.A. et al. Trends in Biochem. Sci. 1982, *1*, 282–286.
    3rd & 4th Seminaires du FFG (French Filtration Group, 1978 and 1979.)

2. Theory and modelling

Skalak, R. et al. Biorheol., 1983, 20, 41–56.

3. Single Erythrocyte Rigidometer (SER)

Kiesewetter, H. et al. Biorheol., 1982, 19, 737–753.
Kiesewetter, H. et al. Scand. J. Clin. Lab. Invest., 1981, *41, Suppl. 156,* 1981.

4. Paper filter methods and 'polymicroviscometry'

Teitel, A. et al. Med. Interna., 1952, 5, 32.
Fahraeus, R. Rheol. Acta, 1961, *1,* 656, 665.
Teitel, P. Nouv. Rev. Fr. Hematol., 1967, *7,* 195–214 and 321–338.
Teitel, P. Blood Cells, 1977, *3,* 55–70.
Staubli, M. et al. Blut, 1979, *39,* 333–344.
Staubli. M. et al. Clin. Hemorheol, 1981, *1,* 341–347.
Staubli. M. et al. Clin. Hemorheol., 1982, *2,* 339–354.
Staubli, M. et al. Schweiz Med Wschr., 1978, *108,* 1593.
Nicolau, C.T. et al. Nature, 1959, *184,* 1808.
Teitel, P. Sangre (Barcelona), 1964, *9,* 421.
Nicolau, C.T. et al. Sangre (Barcelona), 1964, *9,* 282.
Teitel, P. et al. Revue Roumaine de Medecine Interne (Bucharest), 1964, *1,* 223.
Teitel, P. Nature, 1965, *206, 409.*
Teitel, P. Nouvelle Revue Francaise d'Hematologie, 1967, 7, 3.
Teitel, P. et al. Folia Haematologica (Leipzig), 1968, *90,* 281.
Szasz, I. et al. Acta Biochim. Biophys. Acad. Sci. Hungaricae (Budapest), 1970, *5,* 409.
Teitel, P. et al. Haematologia (Budapest), 1971, *5,* 37.
Aspelin, P. et al. Acta Radiologica, 1980, *Suppl. 362,* 127.
Teitel, P. Scand. J. Clin. Lab. Invest., 1981, *41, Suppl. 156,* 235.
Bergents., S.E., et al. Acta Chir. Scand., 1965, *130,* 165–172.
Weed, R.I. et al. JCI, 1968, *48,* 795–809.
Haradin, A.R. et al. Transfusion (Philadelphia), 1969, *9,* 229.
Imre, S. Blut, 1977, *14,* 7.

5. Metal filter methods

Baar, S. Br. J. Haematol., 1976, 34, 69–78.

6. Millipore filter methods

Jandl., J.H. JCl., 1958, 377, 905.
Jandl., J.H. et al. J. Hematol., 1961, *18,* 133.
Ehrly, A.M. et al. Bibl. Anat., 1973, *11,* 55.

7. Nuclepore filter methods

Gregersen, M.L. et al. Science, 1967, *157,* 825.
Usami S. et al. J. Lab. Clin. Med., 1975, *86,* 274–279.
Chien, S., et al. Microvasc. Res., 1971, *3,* 183.
Schmid-Schonbein, H. et al. Blut, 1973, *26,* 369–379.
Lingard, P.S. Microvasc. Res., 1974, *8,* 53–63.
Reid, H. et al. J. Clin. Pathol., 1976, *29,* 855–858.
Lessin, L.S., et al. Blood Cells, 1977, *3,* 241–262.
Johnsson, R. et al. Acta Haematol (Basel), 1978, *60,* 329–340.
Dodds, A.J. et al. Br. Med. J., 1979, *iv,* 1186–1187.
Leblond, P.F. et al. J. Lab. Clin. Med., 1979, *94,* 133–143.
Buchan, P.C. Br. J. Haematol., 1980, *45,* 97–105.
Drummond, M.M. et al. J. Clin. Pathol., 1980, *33,* 373–376.
Norton, J.M. et al. Proc. Soc. Exp. Biol. Med., 1981, *166,* 449–456.
Kenny, M.W. et al. Clin. Hemorheol., 1981, *1,* 135.
Ernst. E.E. et al. Clin. Hemorheol., 1981, *1,* 335–340.
Hanss, M. Biorheol., 1983, *20,* 199–211.
Winkenwerder W. et al. Clin. Hemorheol., 1982, *2,* 201–207.
Slater, N.G.P. et al. Clin. Hemorheol., 1982, *2,* 373–381.
Hanss., M. 4th Semin. du FFG, 1979, 137–153.
Imre. S. Blut., 1977, *34,* 49–52.
Stoltz, J.F. et al. J. Maladies Vacs., 1977, *2,* 37–39.

8. Flow conditions and haemolysis

Chien, S. et al. Microvasc. Res., 1971, *3,* 183–203.
Schmalzer, E.A. et al. Biorheol., 1983, *20,* 29–40.

9. Anticoagulant

Schroer, R. et al. La Ric Clin. Lab., 1981, *ii, Suppl. 1,* 109–116.
Lucas G.S. et al. Clin. Hemorheol., 1984, in press.
Stuart J. et al. Biorheol., 1984, in press.

10. Storage, diurnal variation, ATP depletion

Lucas, G.S. et al. Clin. Hemorheol., 1983, in press.

Weed, R.I. et al. JCI., 1969, *488*, 795–809.

Leterrier, F. *et al.* Clin. Hemorheol., 1983, *3*, *53–95 (comprehensive review.)*.

Nakao K. et al. Nature, 1962, 194, 877–878.

La Celle P.L. Transfusion, 1969, *9*, 238–245.

Deeley, J.O.T. et al. Biochim. Biophys Acta., 1979, 554, 90–101.

Guegen, M. et al. Nouv Presse Med., 1979, 7, 2256–2257.

Sirs, J.A. Blood Cells, 1977, *3*, 409–423.

Feo, C. et al. Blood Cells, 1977, *3*, 153–161.

Genetet, B. et al. 3rd Semin. du FFG, 1978, 11–21.

Meiselman, H.J. et al. Biorheology, 1977, *14*, 11–126.

Meiselman, H.J. et al. Blood, 1978, *52*, 499–504.

Nakao, M. et al. J. Biochem, 1961, *42*, 487–492.

Haradin, A.R. et al. Transfusion (Philadelphia), 1969, *9*, 229.

Hipp, M.J. et al. Transfusion (Philadelphia), 1974, *14*, 447.

Rand, P.W. et al. Clin. Res., 1980, 28, 321A.

Leuenberger, S. et al. VASA, 1983, *11*, 15–20.

Card R.T. et al. Br. J. Haematol., 1983, *53*, 237–240.

Nakashima K. et al. Proc. Natl. Acad. Sci., 1978, *75*, 3823–3825.

Forconi, S. et al. La Ricerca Clin. Lab., 1983, *13*, Suppl. 2, 2777–281.

11. Temperature

Buchan, P.C. Br. J. Haematol, 1980, *45*, 97–105.

Murphy, J.R. J. Lab. Clin. Med., 1967, *69*, 758–775.

Lucas, G.S. et al. Clin. Hemorheol., 1983, in press.

Kikuchi, Y. et al. Experientia, 1982, *38*, 822–824.

Forconi, S. et al. La Ricerca Clin. Lab., 1983, *13*, *Suppl. 2*, 271–276 and 277–281.

Williamson, J.R. et al. Blood, 1975, *46*, 611.

Murphy, J.R. J. Lab. Clin. Med., 1973, *82*, 334–341.

Carlson, D.J. et al. Blood, 1968, *32*, 872–883.

Ham., T.H. et al. Blood, 1968, *32*, 862–871.

Teitel, P. Nature, 1965, *206*, 409.

Karle, J. et al. Scand. J. Clin. Lab. Invest, 1970, *26*, 169.

Schmid-Schönbein, H. et al. Blut, 1973, *26*, 369–279.

12. Haematocrit

Buchan, P.C. Br. J. Haematol., 1980, *45*, 97–105.
Drummond, M.M. et al. J. Clin. Pathol., 1980, *33*, 372–376.
Schmalzer, E.A. et al. Biorheol., 1983, *20*, 28–40.
Rewald, E. et al. Clin. Hemorheol, 1982, *2*, 249–251.

13. MCV/MCH (see also Newborn and Iron deficiency)

Noreton, J.M. et al. Proc. Soc. Exp Biol. Med., 1981, 166.
Slater, N.G.P. et al. Br. J. Haematol., 1982, *2*, 373–381.
Milligan, D.W. et al. Br. J. Haematol., 1982, *50*, 467–473.
Hutton, R.D. Br.J. Haematol., 1979, *43*, 191–199.
Milligan, D.W. et al. Clin. Hemorheol., 1983, *3*, 155–162.
Feo, C. et al. Nouv. Rev. Franc. Hematol., 1982, *24*, 295–299.
Linderkamp, O. et al. Pediatr. Res., 1982, *16*, 964–968.
Linderkamp, O. et al. Pediatr. Res., 1983, *17*, 250–253.
Erslev, A.J. et al. J. Lab. Clin. Med., 1963, *62*, 401–406.
Williams, A.R. et al. Scand. J. Haematol., 1980, *24*, 57–62.

14. White cells

Lichtman, M.A. J. Clin. Invest., 1973, *52*, 350–358.
Lingard, P.S. Microvasc. Res., 1974, *8*, 181.
Alderman, M.J. et al. J. Clin. Pathol., 1981, *34*, 163.
Tanner, L.M. et al. Amer J. Hematol., 1976, *1*, 293–305.
Buchan, P.C. Br. J. Haematol., 1980, *45*, 97–105.
Kenny, M.W. et al. Clin. Hemorheol., 1983, *3*, 191–200.
Milligan, D. Clin. Hemorheol., 1983, *3*, 155–162.
Stuart, J. et al. Clin. Hemorheol., 1983, *3*, 13–21.
Chien, S. et al. Biorheol., 1983, *20*, 11–27.
Schmalzer, E.A. et al. Biorheol., 1983, *20*, 29–40.
Lucas, G.S. et al. Clin. Hemorheol., 1983, in press.
Slater, N.G.P. et al. Clin. Hemorheol., 1982, *2*, 373–281.

15. Platelets

Schroer, R. et al. La Ric. Clin. Lab., 1981, *11*, Suppl. 1, 109–116.

16. Plasma and plasma proteins

Kenny, M.M. et al. Clin. Hemorheol., 1981, *1*, 135–146.

Winkenwerder, W. et al. Clin. Hemorheol., 1982, *2*, 201–207.
Ernst, E. et al. Clin. Hemorheol., 1983, *3*, 31–36.
Koyama, T. et al. Biorheol., 1982, *19*, 579–585.
Buchan, P.C. Br. J. Haematol., 1980, *45*, 97–105.

17. Suspending medium

Chien, S. Blood Cells, 1977, *3*, 71–99.
Kenny, M.W. et al. Clin. Hemorheol, 1981, *1*, 135–146.

18. Calcium

O'Rear, E.A. et al. Biochim. Biophys. Acta., 1982, *691*, 274–280.
Rogausch, H. Pflugers Arch., 1978, *373*, 43–47.

19. pH, pO2, pCO2

Buchan, P.C. Br. J. Haematol., 1980, *45*, 97–105.
Murphy, J.R. J. Lab. Clin. Med., 1967, *69*, 758–775.
Norton, J.M. et al. Proc. Soc. Exp. Biol. Med., 1981, 166, 449–456.
Kikuchy, Y. et al. Experientia, 1979, 35, 343–344.
LaCelle, P.L. et al. JCI, 1970, 49, 54A–55A.
Smith, B.D. et al. Blood, 1979, 53, 15–18.
Burnard, E. et al. Bibl. Haematol., 1968, 29, 1155.
Schmid-Schönbein, H. et al. Blut, 1973, *26*, 369–379.

20. Osmolarity

Slater, N.G.P. et al. Clin. Hemorheol., 1982, *2*, 373–381.
Buchan, P.C. Br. J. Haematol., 1980, *45*, 97–105.
Feo, C. et al. Nouv Rev. Franc Hematol., 1982, *24*, 295–299.
Ham, T.H. et al. Blood, 1968, 847–861.

21. Sickle cell disease

Chien, S. et al. J. Clin. Invest., 1970, *49*, 623–634.
Usami, S. et al. J. Lab. Clin. Med. 1975, *86*, 274–282.
Lessin, L.S. et al. Blood Cells, 1977, *3*, 241–262.
Usami, S. et al. Microvasc. Res., 1975, *9*, 324–334.
Chien, S. et al. Blood Cells, 1977, *3*, 283–296.
Messer, M.J. et al. JCI Med., 1970, *76*, 537–547.
Ohnishi, S.T. Blood Cells, 1982, *8*, 79–87.

Serjeant, B.E. et al. Br. J. Ophthalmol., 1983, in press.
Hipp, M.J. et al. Transfusion (Philadelphia), 1974, *14*, 447.
Gulley, M.L. et al. AM. J. Hematol., 1982, *13*, 283–291.
Kenny, M.W. et al. Br J. Haematol., 1981, *49*, 103–109.
Kenny, M.W. et al. Br. J. Haematol., 1983, *55*, 465–471.
Serjeant, B.E. et al. Br. J. Haematol., 1983, *55*, 479–486.

22. Other haemolytic anaemias

Jandl, J.H. et al. J. Hematol., 1961, *18*, 133.
Miller, L. et al. Am. J. Trop. Med. Hygiene, 1972, *21*, 133–137.

Murphy, J.R. J. Lab. Clin. Med., 1967, *69*, 758–725.
Johnsson, R. et al. Acta Haematol (Basel), 1978, *60*, 329–340.
Leblond, P.F. et al. J. Lab. Clin. Med., 1979, *94*, 133.
Miller, L.H. et al. JCl., 1971, *50*, 1451–1455.
Brereton, W. et al. J. Lab. Clin. Med., 1974, *83*, 112–118.
LaCelle, P.L. Semin. Haematol., 1970, *7*, 355–371.
Teitel, P. et al. Biorheol, 1972, *9*, 164–165.
Marik, T. et al. Vnitr. Lek., 1980, *26*, 1079–1085.
Teitel, P. et al. Nouv. Rev. Fr. Hematol., 1967, *7*, 321–338.
Tillmann, W. et al. Br. J. Haematol, 1979, *43*, 401–411.
Nicolau, C.T. et al. Sangre, 1964, *9*, 282–286.
Bessis, M. et al. Blood Cells, 1975, *1*, 315–321.
Allard, C. et al. Blood Cells, 1977, *19*, 209–221.
Bessis, M. Nouv. Rev. Fr. Hematol., 1977, *28*, 75–94.
Leblond, P.F. et al. Br. J. Haematol., 1978, *39*, 63–70.
Mohandas, N. et al. Semin. Hematol., 1979, *16*, 95–114.
Nakashima, K. et al. Blood, 1979, *53*, 481–485.
Schroter, W. et al. Br. J. Haematol., 1977, *36*, 475–484.
Winstein, R.S. et al. Toxicol. Appl. Pharmacol, 1975, *32*, 545–558.
Teitel, P. Sangre, 1964, *9*, 421–429.
Brabec, V. Folia Haematologica (Leipzig), 1976, *103*, 552.
Jocobasch, G. et al. Studia Biophysica, 1982, *90*, 115–117.

23. Iron deficiency

Slater, N.G.P. et al. Clin. Hemorheol., 1982, *2*, 373–381.
Tillman, W. et al. Blut, 1980, *40*, 179–186.
Cazrd, R.T. et al. Blood, 1971, *37*, 725–732.
Milligan, D.W. et al. Br. J. Haematol., 1982, *50*, 467–473.
Milligan, D.W. Clin. Hemorheol., 1983, *3*, 155–162.

24. Other blood disorders

Megaloblastic anaemia
Ballas, S.K. et al. Am. J. Clin. Pathol., 1976, *66*, 953–957.

Polycythaemia
Rewald, E. et al. Br. J. Haematol., 1981, *47*, 485.
Milligan, D.W. Clin. Hemorheol., 1983, *3*, 155–162.
Hutton, R.D. Br. J. Haematol., 1979, *43*, 191–199.
(Fallots) Naknche, M. et al. Clin. Hemorheol., 1983, *3*, 177–189.

Splenectomy
Robertson, D.A.F. et al. Br. Med. J. 1981, *283*, 573–578.

25. Renal diseases and dialysis

Rosenmund, A. et al. Ann. Int Med., 1975, *82*, 460–465.
Inauen, W. et al. Europ. J. Clin. Invest., 1982, *12*, 173–176.
Kikuchi, Y. et al. Nephron, 1982, *30*, 8–14.
Forman, S. et al. Ann Int. Med., 1973, *79*, 841–843.
Mathe, P. 3rd Semin. du FFG, 1978, 295–299.
Renaud, M. et al. 4th Semin du FFG, 1979, 395–410.
Simon, P. et al. 3rd Semin du FFG, 1978, 339–342.
Rosenmund, A. et al. Schweiz. Med. Wschr, 1974, *104*, 1394.

26. Alcohol and liver diseases

Garnier, M. et al. Clin. Hemorheol., 1983, *3*, 45–52.
Hanss, M. et. al. Path. Biol., 1981, *29*, 496–498.
Boivin, P. et al. Ann Int. Med., 1971, *122*, 467–477.
Rogausch, H. Acta Haematol., 1971, *46*, 211–220.

27. Injury, burns, surgery, anaesthesia, radiation

Extracorporeal circulation
Starling, J.R. et al. Surgery, 1975, *77*, 562–568.
Vanuxem, D. et al. Clin. Hemorheol., 1983, *3*, 163–175.
Ohshima, N. Biorheol., 1978, 15, 295–302.

Surgery
Dodds, A.J. et al. Thrombos. Res., 1980, *18*, 561–565.
Ernst, E. et al. Scand. J. Clin. Lab. Invest., 1981, *41*, *Suppl. 156*, 317–319.

Sirs, J.A. et al. Thromb. Res., 1974, *5,* 657–666.

Burns
Guimbretriere, J. et al. 3rd Semin du FFG, 1978, 301–317.
Baar, S. Clin. Chim. Acta., 1979, *94,* 181–189.
Baar, S. Burns, 1976, *3,* 46–59.
Braasch, D. et al. Pflugers Arch., 1971, *323,* 41–49.
Guimbretriere, J. et al. 4th Semin du FFG, 1979, 313–324.
Schachar, N.S. et al. Can. J. Surg., 1974, *17,* 239–243.
Baar, S. Br. J. Exp. Pathol., 1982, *63,* 644–650.

Injury
Bergentz, S. et al. Acta Chir. Scand., 1965, *130,* 165–172.

Radiation
Karle, H. et al. Scand. J. Haematol., 1971, *8,* 72.

fo11Anaesthesia
Baker, R. et al. Progr. Clin. Biol. Res., 1975, *1,* 437–453.
Chen, R.Y.Z. et al. Anesthesiology, 1979, *51,* 245–250.
De Bruijne, A.W. et al. Biochem. Pharmacol., 1979, *28,* 177–182.
Drummond, A.R. et al. In: Stoltz, J.F., Drouin, P. (eds). Hemorheology
and Diseases. Paris, Doin Editeurs, 1980, pp. 445–450.
Palek, J. et al. Blood, 1977, *50,* 155–164.
Van Gastel, L.F.J. et al. Biochem. Biophys. Res. Comm., 1973, *55,* 1240–
1245.

28. Venous thromboembolism

Lowe, G.D.O. et al. Lancet, 1982, *i,* 409–412.
Leroy, J. et al. 3rd Seminaire du FFG, 1978, 331–337.

29. Coronary artery disease

Dodds, A.J. et al. Br. Heart J., 1980, *44,* 508–511.
Drummond, M.M. et al. J. Clin. Pathol., 1980, *33,* 373–376.
Forconi, S. et al. La Ricerca Clin. Lab., 1983, *13, Suppl. 2,* 195–208.
Botas, L. et al. Acta. Med. Portuguesa, 1983, *4 (Suppl.),* 87–89.

30. Cerebrovascular disease

Lorient-Roudant, M.F. et al. Scand. J. Clin. Lab. Invest., 1981, *41,* Suppl.
156, 203–208.

Lorient, M.F. et al. La Semaine Hop Paris, 1979, *55,* 27–30.
Boisseau, M.R. et al. 3rd Semin du FFG, 1978, 229–243.
Boisseau, M.R. et al. 4th Semin du FFG, 1979, 273–287.
Fedin, A.L. et al. Zh. Nevropatol Psikhiat., 1978, *78,* 1627–1635.
Gousser, El et al. Zh. Nevropatol. Psikhiat., 1978, *78,* 1798–1804.
Terrier, M. Tonus, 1979, *429, 18–19.*
Ionescu, D.A. et al. Blut, 1979, 39, 351.
Palareti, G. et al. Int. Angiol., 1983, *2,* 179–183.

31. Peripheral arterial disease

Ehrly, A.M. et al. Vasa, 1976, *5,* 319–322.
Reid, H.L. et al. Lancet, 1976, *i,* 666–668.
Drummond, M.M. et al. J. Clin. Pathol., 1980, *33,* 373–376.
Alderman, M.J. et al. J. Clin. Pathol., 1981, *34,* 163.
Stuart, J. et al. Clin. Hemorheol., 1983, *3,* 23–30.
Dormandy, J.A. et al. J. Physiol., 1978, *275,* 19–20.
Perego, M.A. et al. Angeiologie, 1981, *33,* 137–146.
Bidet, J.M. et al. Scand. J. Clin. Invest., 1981, *41, Suppl. 156,* 189–191.
Angelkort, B. et al. J. Int. Med. Res., 1980, *8,* 242–246.
Winkenwender, W. et al. Clin. Hemorheol., 1982, *2,* 201–207.
Perego, M.A. et al. LaRicerca Clin. Lab., 1981, *11 Suppl. 1,* 281–291.
Ehrly, A.M. et al. Scand. J. Clin. Lab. Invest., 1981, *41, Suppl. 156,* 181–
    184.
Goebel, K.M. et al. Schweiz Med. Wochenschr., 1981, *111,* 1538.

32. Raynaud's syndrome

Dodds, A.J. et al. Br. Med. J. 1979, *iv,* 1186–1187.
Dowd, P.M. et al. Br. Med., J., 1981, *283,* 350.
Dintenfass, L. Angiol., 1977, *128,* 472–481.
Merlen, J.F. et al. 3rd Semin du FFG, 1978, 319–329.
Sarteel A.M. et al. 4th Semin du FFG, 1979, 305–312.

33. Diabetes

McMillan, D.E. et al. Diabetes, 1978, 27, 895–901.
Schmid-Schönbein, H. et al. Diabetes, 1976, *25,* 897–902.
Barnes, A.J. et al. Lancet, 1977, *ii,* 789–791.
Stuart, J. et al. Clin. Hemorheol, 1983, *3,* 23–30.
Neumann, V. et al. Clin. Hemorheol, 1983, *3,* 13–21.
Juhan, I. et al. Lancet, 1982, *i,* 535–537.

Juhan, I. et al. Marseille Medical, 1978, *155*, 21–23.

Rand, P.W. et al. Clin. Hemorheol., 1981, *1*, 373–384.

Pozza, G. et al. La Ricerca Clin. Lab., 1981, *11*, *Suppl. 1*, 317–126.

Juhan, I. et al. Nouv. Presse. Med., 1981, *10*, 910–918.

Le Dehevat, C. et al. 4th Semin du FFG, 1979, 99–115.

Le Dehevat, C. et al. 3rd Semin du FFG, 1978, 147–186 and 259–272.

Renaudin, J.M. et al. 3rd Semin du FFG, 1978, 281–294.

Coccheri, S. et al. J. Int. Med. Res., 1982, *10*, 394–398.

Carandente, O. et al. Acta Diabet. Lat., 1982, *19*, 359–368.

Sewchand, L.S. et al. Microcirculation, 1981/82, *1*, 361–380.

Bidet, J.M. et al. 4th Semin du FFG, 1979, 227–235.

Juhan, I., et al. Nouv Presse. Med, 1978, *7*, 759.

Juhan, I. et al. Nouv. Rev. Franc. Hematol., 1979, *21*, *Suppl. 1*, 61.

Juhan, I. et al. 3rd Semin. du FFG, 1978, 135–145.

Juhan, I. et al. 4th Semin du FFG, 1979, 219–226.

Knight, K. et al. Biorheol, 1978, 15, 51–52.

Le Devehat, C. et al. Ann. Biol. Clin., 1978, *56*, 530.

Le Devehat, C et al. 4th Semin du FFG, 1979, 99–177.

Stoltz, J.F et al. 4th Semin. du FFG, 1979, 251–272.

Bryszewska, M. et al. Diabetologia, 1983, *24*, 311–313.

Vague, P. et al. Diabetes, 1982, *32*, *Suppl. 2*, 88–91.

Levy-Cruz, F. et al. Acta Med. Portuguesa, 1983, *4*, *(Suppl.)* 83–85.

Juhan, I. et al. Nouv. Presse. Med., 1979, *50*, 4083–4086.

Juhan, I. et al. Scand. J. Clin. Lab. Invest., 1981, *41*, *Suppl. 156*, 159–164.

Juhan, I. et al. Clin. Hemorheol., 1983, *3*, 266.

Juhan, I. et al. Clin. Hemorheol., 1983, *3*, 316.

34. Lipid disorders

Shiga, T. et al. Clin. Hemorheol., 1982, 2, 77–84.

Lowe, G.D.O. et al. Lancet, 1982, *1*, 472–475.

Garnier, M. et al. Clin. Hemorheol., 1983, *3*, 45–52.

35. Hypertension

Dintenfass, L. et al. Haemostasis, 1978, *7*, 298–362.

Freitas, J. et al. Acta Med. Portuguesa, 1983, *4*, *(Suppl.)*, 77–78.

Carlota Proenca, M. et al. Acta Med. Portuguesa, 1983, *4*, *(Suppl.)*,
79–80, and 81–82.

36. Smoking

Lowe, G.D.O. et al. In: Stoltz, J.F., Droin, P. eds. Hemorheology and Diseases. Paris: Doin Editeurs, 1980, pp. 349–352.

Norton, J.M. et al. Blood, 1981, *57*, 671–674.

Lagrue, G. et al. Nouv. Pr Med., 1979, *8*, 4079–4081.

Landgraf, H. et al. Clin. Hemorheol, 1981, *3*, 241–249.

Ehrly, A.M. et al. Herz/Kreislauf, 1978, *10*, 245–246.

Grigoleit, H.G. et al. Dtsch. Med. Wschr., 1978, *103*, 339–341.

Frietas, J. Acta Med. Portuguesa, 1983, *4*, *(Suppl.)*, 73–75.

37. Age

Perego, M.A. et al. Giorn. Geront., 1981, *29*, 560–564.

Terranova, R. et al. La Ricerca Clin. Lab., 1981, *11*, 345–352.

Gueguen, M. et al. 4th Seminaire de FFG, 1979, 898–98.

Imre, S. et al. Acta Physiol Acad. Sci. Hung., 1979, *53*, 23–30.

38. Sex, pill, menstrual cycle

Grumel, J.M. Med. Actuelle, 1976, *3*, 10.

Leroy-Deval, et al. 3rd Seminaire du FFG, 1978, 191–200.

Mercke, C. et al. Ann Int. Med., 1976, *85*, 322–324.

Oski, F.A. et al. Ann Int. Med., 1972, *77*, 417–419.

Warniez, C. et al. Rev. Fr. Gynecol. Obstet., 1977, *72*, 141–145.

Durocher, J.R. et al. Proc. Soc. Exp. Biol. Med., *150*, 368–371.

39. Pregnancy and disorders

Buchan, P.C. Br. J. Haematol., 1980, *45*, 97–105.

Stuart, J. et al. Br. J. Haematol., 1983, *53*, 353–355.

Thorburn, et al. Br J. Obstet. Gyneacol., 1982, *89*, 117–122.

Inglis, T.C.M. et al. Br. J. Haematol., 1982, *50*, 461–465.

Zondervan, H.A. et al. Eur. J. Obstet. Gynecol. Reprod. Biol., 1982, *13*, 389.

Gresele, P. et al. Br. J. Haematol., 1982, *52*, 340–342.

Heilmann, L. et al. Blut, 1977, *35*, 213–221.

Durocher, J.R. et al. Proc. Soc. Exp. Biol. Med., 1975, *150*, 368–371.

40. Newborn

Buchan, P.C. Br. J. Haematol., 1980, *45*, 97–105.

Tillman, W. et al. Blut, 1977, *34,* 281–288.

Gross, G.P. et al. Pediatr. Res., 1972, *6,* 593–599.

Bergquist, G. et al. Bibl. Anat., 1977, *16,* 510–512.

Linderkamp, O. et al. Clin. Hemorheol., 1981, *1,* 575–584.

Coulombel, L. et al. Biol. Neonate, 1982, *42, 284–290.*

Delobel, J. et al. 4th Seminar du Groupe de Travail sur La Filtration Erythrocytaire, 1979, 77–87.

Feo, C. Nouv. Rev. Franc Hematol., 1979, 21, Suppl. 1, 60.

Gaehtgens, P. et al. Bibl. Anat., 1974, *13,* 107–108.

Linderkamp, O. et al. Pediatr. Res., 1983, *17,* 250–253.

Grigoleit, H.G. et al. Dtsch. Med. Wschr., 1978, *103,* 339–341.

41. Miscellaneous

Myopathies
Beyer, P. et al. Nouv. Presse. Med., 1977, *6,* 1663.

Delaunay, J. et al. Nouv. Presse. Med., 1977, *6,* 1129–1136.

Matheson, D.W. et al. Science, 1974, *184,* 165–166.

Percy, A.K. et al. Nature, 1975, *258,* 147–148.

Somer, H. et al. Neurology, 1979, *29,* 519–522.

Johnsson, R. et al. J. Neurol. Sci., 1983, *58,* 399–407.

Neurology
Sills, R.H., et al. J. Pediatr., 1982, *101,* 395–398. (Meningitis).

Butterfield, D.A. et al. Biochim. Biophys. Acta, 1979, *551,* 452–458. (Huntington's chorea).

Pollock, S. et al. J. Neurol. Neurosurg. Psychiat., 1982, *45,* 762–770. (Multiple sclerosis).

Thyroid disease
Wardrop, C. et al. Lancet, 1969, *i,* 1243.

Lorient, M.F. et al. 4th Semin du FFG, 1979, 325–332.

Lorient-Roudunt, M.F. et al. Med Hyg., 1982, *40,* 4375–4378.

Infections
Staubli, M. et al. Schweiz Med Wschr., 1979, *109,* 1903.

Miller, L.H. et al. Am. J. Trop. Med. Hyg., 1972, *21,* 133–137.

Lee, M.V. et al. J. Med., 1982, *13,* 479–485.

Cancer
Cohen, M.H. J. Nat Cancer Inst., 1979, *63,* 525–526.

98

Racing
    Reinhart, W.H. et al. J. Appl. Physiol., 1983, *54*, 827–830.

Altitude
    Palareti, G. et al. Angiology, 1984, in press.

Commentary

M. Verstraete

What could be the purpose of inviting a non-expert to the inner circle of highly specialised scientists united by a common glossary of terms, divided by their personal techniques, haunted by red cells intimately mixed in their suspension with white cells, platelets, endothelial cells and their respective products – a group in search of a clinical counterpart for the observed in vitro haemorheological findings? One plausible explanation is my long acquaintance with many of this friendly group; I rather suspect our shrewd chairman wants the cold gaze of a non-committed, interested observer and some provocative remarks.

I was amazed to notice that at a meeting of fundamental haemorheologists, attention is shifting away from plasma or whole blood viscosity towards red cell deformability. The disenchantment comes when glaring to the magnificent and so expensive haemoviscosity meters, one realizes the enormous technical difficulties prevailing in assessing in a practical and reliable way either phenomenon. Methodological problems obviously are still dominating the masters of thought and mathematical methods. There is also a controversy, if not divergence of opinion, on some basic principles how to measure red cell filtration, as three types of systems are used: constant flow rate systems with measurements of pressure increase, constant pressure systems with measurements of volume flow rate, and variable pressure systems with measurement of volume flow rates. The impact of the blood sampling, handling and storage techniques, the effects of haematocrit, leucocytes, platelets and plasma constituents on filtration tests, and the importance of the filters or microsieves used all appear to be bewildering problems to an outsider. There is, therefore, less surprise that the coefficient of variation of each of the methods proposed remains exceedingly high (up to 30%), even when the tests are performed in a centre of rheological excellence.

A similar embarrassing period of technical vaguery and methodological uncertainty has beset any new branch of medical science and will eventually also in haemorheology find a suitable solution. One wonders whether in the meantime more energy should not be invested by some in comparing simultaneously several methods, as it is increasingly apparent that each is recognizing different rheological features. Indeed, data obtained with one method cannot be equated with those obtained by another one. For the time being it may be rewarding to concentrate also on the wood, even at the expense of the individual trees. Inevitably, clinicians are tempted to look at clinical conditions through relatively imperfect tools; one feels uneasy, however, hearing that changes in rheological parameters can be observed in most divergent pathological situations, as, for example, neurological patients with a minor infarcted area in the brain, in patients with Prinzmetal-angina, diabetes, hypertension and multiple sclerosis. It is likely that the medical community would rather be critical to the interpretation of rheological tests with such a low specificity and tend to consider their results as mainly influenced by one of the numerous acute phase reactions or longer-term stress response. After all, filterability tests are not measuring a real property of red cells but rather their performance or behaviour in a very artificial situation (e.g. using in vitro shear stresses two magnitudes higher than in vivo). Making filtration tests increasingly more sensitive to subtle changes in red cell deformability may be compromising specificity.

There are a few questions which may help to point towards clinical relevance of haemorheological studies. Is there a quantitative relationship between the changes in rheological parameters and the severity of a clinical condition (chronic state), and how do they behave at times of rapid clinical deterioration or improvement? Do haemorheological parameters really have a prognostic value as was suggested, e.g., in diabetic microangiopathy and stroke? As was adequately stressed during this meeting when exploring clinical conditions, the same haemorheological studies should also be applied in an appropriate control group, particularly as clinicians are confronted with discrete or small changes which, in the absence of other abnormalities, are well tolerated.

It appears to me that as long as instruments and methodology used in clinical haemorheology are not better standardised and more precise information is secured on the clinical relevance of the results obtained, it would be premature to embark in a long-term intervention study. In missing the right boat, a new opportunity may not come again in the next decade.

Concluding remarks

P. Gaehtgens

The activity of this group at this year's meeting and the previous meetings represents an attempt to improve and analyse the usefulness of a very specific method to determine an at least theoretically well-defined property of the red cells. If I think back to the previous meetings and compare where we are after these two days with where we were when we started, I think we have not entirely been unsuccessful. A few years ago there were so many different factors which could potentially influence the result of a filtration measurement that it took the efforts of a number of laboratories to look into the details of this method. At this stage we have achieved at least a satisfying conclusion as to which factors are more important and which are not. If I may remind you that when we met last time everybody was very concerned about the effect of white cells on the filtration test. This problem may have been solved, since we now know how to effectively remove white cells, and then measure what we originally intended to measure, namely red cell filterability rather than blood filterability. The intention of measuring the filterability of blood was to be able to quantitatively say something about red cell properties. We have excluded certain factors which introduced errors into the measurement. At the time of the London Clinical Haemorheology meeting there were more warnings than recommendations. I think now we have more recommendations than warnings. For instance, the problem of anticoagulation is much clearer now than it was two years ago: if you use short storage times you can use either heparin or EDTA but if you have to wait for longer times then you may be allowed only to use EDTA. There are a number of problems which indeed this group has solved, and I think this should be mentioned.

On the other hand, there are also a few problems remaining, for instance the problem of temperature. One member of the group suggested that even the patient should be kept at a defined temperature if the measurement is to be reproducible! The standardisation of the filter itself still presents a problem. As Professor Verstraete rightly said, as long as the coefficient of variation is as large as it is in the method commonly used, it is not very likely that we are going to detect more subtle changes which may in the very end be relevant in the in vivo situation. I think it is in general important to realise that red cell deformability has many facets, and therefore it is justified to conclude that if we want to learn more about the situation in which the red cell spends its lifetime, or about the effect of an alteration of the cell's properties, then we have to use more than one method. Focussing on filterability is just picking out one of these aspects. And in this sense I think the second part of today's meeting really opened up the scope of the group, because here we were discussing a strategy for also measuring other haemorheological parameters in addition to the one property that we have looked at in the beginning. Here, the 'profile' approach may be valuable. It seems, however, that many of the other methods which we have not discussed require a similar discussion as the one conducted on filterability in this group, because there are almost as many problems inherent in those methods as there are in filtration measurements.

I will not close this meeting without extending all of our thanks to those who in the background and at the front have organised this meeting, particularly Barbara Komoniewska. Thank you all very much.